A DASH *of* Aloha

HEALTHY HAWAI'I CUISINE AND LIFESTYLE

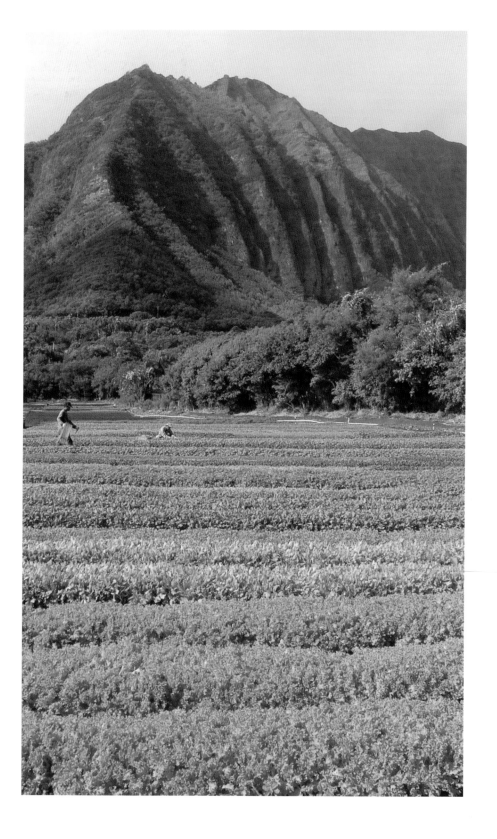

A DASH *of* Aloha

HEALTHY HAWAI'I CUISINE AND LIFESTYLE

KAPI'OLANI COMMUNITY COLLEGE
University of Hawai'i

WATERMARK
PUBLISHING

Kapiʻolani Community College is an
Equal Opportunity/Affirmative Action Institution.

The research and development of the recipes, the nutritional
analysis, and staffing for the publication of this book is funded
by a grant from the U.S. Department of Agriculture / CSREES.

Funding for the printing and publication of this book
was provided by the HMSA Foundation.

ISBN 978-0-9796769-4-9

Library of Congress Control Number:
2007941619

Watermark Publishing
1088 Bishop Street, Suite 310
Honolulu, HI 96813
Telephone: Toll-free 1-866-900-BOOK
Web site: www.bookshawaii.net
e-mail: sales@bookshawaii.net

Printed in Korea

Table of Contents

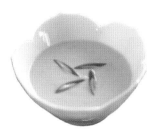

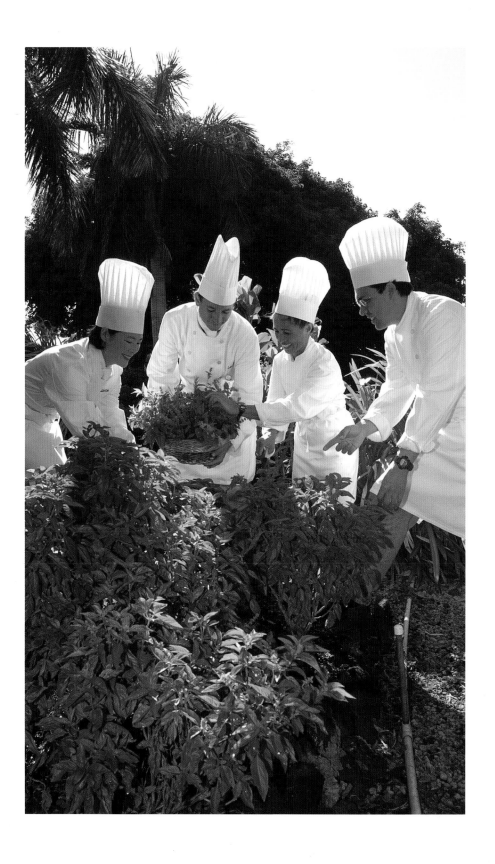

Foreword

The Culinary Arts Department at Kapi'olani Community College (KCC), one of seven Culinary Institute of the Pacific education centers within the University of Hawai'i community college system, is proud to present this healthy Hawai'i cuisine and activity book based on the Dietary Approach to Stop Hypertension (DASH) eating plan. Over the past few years, students of cooking classes, patrons of KCC's Ka 'Ikena Restaurant and the general public have inquired about how to cook and eat healthy. In response, we utilized a grant from the U.S. Department of Agriculture / Cooperative State Research, Education and Extension Service (USDA / CSREES) to conduct research and nutritional analysis of recipes created by Hawai'i chefs. Their recipes, which include local farm products, are an exciting collection of dishes that highlight the best of what Hawai'i's agriculture offers—vibrant, colorful produce with uniquely intense flavors cultivated by the Islands' climate and rich soil. The Hawai'i Medical Service Association (HMSA) provided a generous grant to assist in the publication and printing of this book.

KCC's dietitian, exercise specialist, food photographer and team of culinary instructors enthusiastically embrace this plan for healthy lifestyles that combines good eating habits and regular physical activity. We strongly believe that all foods should be enjoyed, with moderation. Instead of counting every calorie of every meal, it's more critical to learn how to balance the nutritional value in each dish over periods of days and weeks. Equally important is creating tasty variations in order to get the maximum enjoyment out of preparing and eating our daily meals, rather than stressing over calories and embarking on fad diets.

We are very fortunate to have the help of several key partners in this project. We want to thank the staffs of the National Kidney Foundation of Hawai'i and the American Heart Association of Hawai'i for their invaluable advice and contribution to this book. Hawai'i's farmers, fishermen and ranchers are also indispensable, as through their toils and labor they provide us with the building blocks for our gourmet creations. The Hawai'i Farm Bureau Federation's farmers markets and the historical Honolulu Chinatown markets literally bring these flavorful products much closer to our homes, making eating fresh so much easier.

So with a DASH of Aloha, we wish you good health, and *bon appetit*!

Ronald K. Takahashi, M.B.A., CFBE, CHE
Chairperson, Culinary Arts Department
Kapi'olani Community College
UNIVERSITY OF HAWAI'I

The HMSA Foundation is pleased to present *A DASH of Aloha* in collaboration with Kapi'olani Community College and its Culinary Institute of the Pacific. This unique cookbook features healthy recipes that explore the flavors of Pacific Rim cultures and take advantage of fresh produce grown here in Hawai'i. We hope these recipes help you make healthy choices that are easy, interesting and attractive. As we all know, good nutrition is an important component of a healthy lifestyle for yourself and your 'ohana.

For many years, the HMSA Foundation has supported programs that promote good nutrition. We are proud to partner with the Culinary Institute of the Pacific on this project and hope you enjoy these creative and tasty recipes.

Cliff K. Cisco
Vice President
HMSA Foundation

I am pleased to have the opportunity to partner with our colleagues at Kapiʻolani Community College, University of Hawaiʻi, to provide information to the world about Hawaiʻi's tasty and healthy recipes, local foods and dishes. In Hawaiʻi we have a rich ethnic heritage and a unique fusion of dishes. We value our local, tropical Island foods. Ron Takahashi and the Kapiʻolani Community College Culinary Arts Department have been leaders and collaborators in providing a tasty and healthy food environment.

Every day we eat. We want healthy and tasty foods. Eating is one of life's necessities and one of life's pleasures. We make choices from a myriad of foods and dishes. The DASH eating plan has been shown to promote health and prevent disease among U.S. Mainland populations. The DASH eating plan has been adopted by national organizations as a recommended food pattern. *A DASH of Aloha* is an elegant display of how our local foods and dishes can be tasty and also be incorporated into a healthy DASH eating plan.

I am proud to contribute to this effort to celebrate Hawaiʻi's food diversity and to share it with others. We can share aloha, be healthy and enjoy food by surrounding ourselves with fresh, healthy cuisine.

With a Dash of Aloha,

Rachel Novotny, Ph.D., R.D.
Professor, Nutrition, *University of Hawaiʻi*
Director, *Kaiser Permanente Center for Health Research Hawaiʻi*

The Culinary Arts Department
Kapiʻolani Community College

The Culinary Arts Department at Kapiʻolani Community College is one of seven unique culinary education centers of **The Culinary Institute of the Pacific (CIP)** within the University of Hawaiʻi system, located on the islands of Oʻahu, Maui, Hawaiʻi and Kauaʻi. The CIP's mission is to offer Hawaiʻi, and the global community, training and education in all aspects of the culinary arts.

The premier CIP center on Oʻahu is located at Kapiʻolani Community College, nestled on the slopes of Diamond Head Crater, overlooking the Pacific Ocean and Waikīkī. Accredited by the American Culinary Federation (ACF), the campus offers a world-class learning environment that includes 10 instructional kitchens, and a 130-seat demonstration auditorium, as well as on-campus restaurants and banquet rooms. The CIP excels in interna-

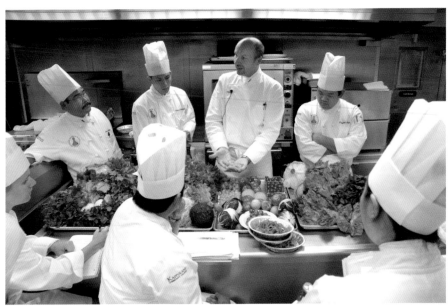

Associate Professor Frank Leake teaching Fundamentals of Cookery class.

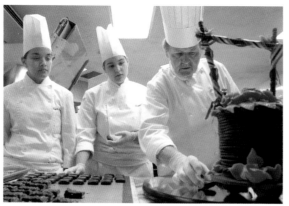
Pastry Arts Professor Ernst Hiltbrand demonstrates for students.

tionalizing its culinary education program, blending the techniques, traditions and influences of Asia and the Pacific with the classical styles of Europe and American cuisine. The Institute's faculty is composed of award-winning chefs, plus food and beverage experts, many of whom are graduates of the Culinary Institute of America, Le Cordon Bleu, Johnson & Wales University and Kapiʻolani Community College.

The **Ka ʻIkena Restaurant** at Kapiʻolani Community College is operated by students from the Culinary Arts Department and is open to the public. Throughout the year, a variety of cuisines are served for lunch and dinner.

For folks in the community who love to cook (and eat), Kapiʻolani Community College offers **non-credit continuing education classes** to the public on Saturdays, plus some weeknights. Basic culinary skills and home-style cuisines from around the world are taught by professional chef instructors and culinary specialists. The program also offers culinary tours of Island farms and foreign culinary destinations.

The public is also welcome to visit **The Kulia Grill** at the John A. Burns School of Medicine at Kakaʻako. It is operated by the Culinary Arts Department's staff, where healthy menu items are showcased daily.

CONTACT INFORMATION

Ka ʻIkena Restaurant reservations: 734-9499
Non-credit Classes: 734-9441
Culinary Tours: 734-9473

Kapiʻolani Community College: 734-9484
Culinary Arts Department
4303 Diamond Head Road,
Honolulu, HI 96816
www.kcc.hawaii.edu/object/culinaryarts.html

Dining at the Ka ʻIkena Restaurant and
220 Grill at Kapiolani Community College
— www.kcc.hawaii.edu/page/dining

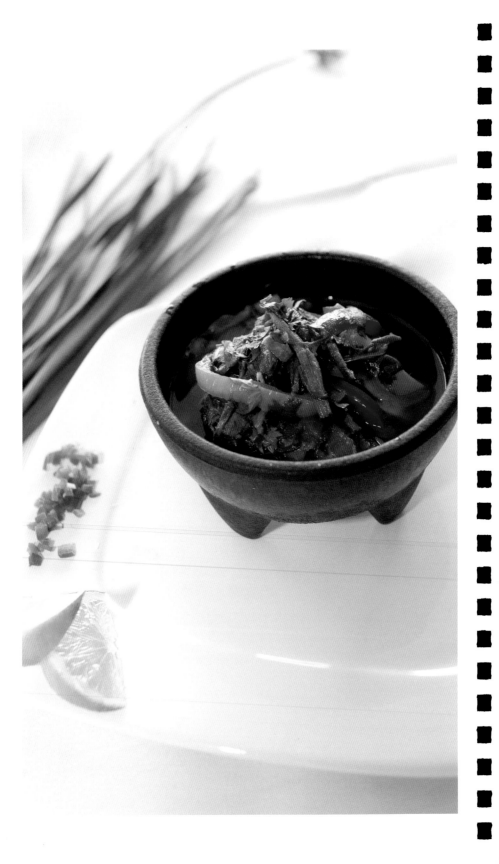

Chapter 1

Eat Well, Eat Healthy
How to use this DASH
"not just a cookbook" book

Daniel Leung, A.S. (Culinary Arts), M.S.W.
Educational Specialist
Kapiʻolani Community College

If you find counting calories and sticking to an exercise regimen difficult, this book is for you! You can eat well, and eat healthy … really.

This book is about eating, not dieting. It is about variations, not restrictions. It is by no means definitive. This is just a starting point—guidelines and ideas with which you can experiment, explore and create your own recipes with your favorite ingredients. We want you to think outside the bento box. We want you to eat farm fresh, not factory processed.

Our goal is to show you how to improve your health by eating delicious meals. It is designed to introduce the major concepts emphasized in the easy-to-use DASH (Dietary Approach to Stop Hypertension) eating and activity plan, and give you the tools to get started. Above all, we want you to eat well. Often, we associate eating healthy with bland food, sacrifice and uninspiring dishes. Not so in this book. We demonstrate how to use locally-grown, farm-fresh ingredients to excite your palate and bring zest to your meals. Furthermore, the examples of recipes and ingredients will help you follow the eating plan without having to count every single calorie or milligram of sodium at every meal. Realistically, who can count calories and the milligrams at every meal, every day? Drastic fad dieting can upset your sense of well-being, which makes it difficult to maintain your overall enjoyment of food. The DASH eating plan includes fresh, flavorful foods that everyone enjoys, and makes it easy to keep up healthy eating habits.

The DASH eating plan describes a set of goals for you to achieve over time.
For certain meals, on certain days, you may eat more than the recommended servings of a food or exceed the recommended limit of sodium, saturated fat or cholesterol in just one dish. Don't stress about it. As long as you pay attention to the average amount you are consuming over time, you can easily stay within the overall limit. You should use the recipes in this book, along with their nutritional facts, not to limit you, but to guide you toward an overall goal of health and well-being.

What is the DASH eating plan?

The National Heart, Lung, and Blood Institute (NHLBI) developed the Dietary Approach to Stop Hypertension (DASH) eating plan. It's based on scientific studies that show that blood pressure is reduced with meals that are low in saturated fat, cholesterol and total fat. The DASH eating plan emphasizes eating fruits, vegetables and fat-free or low-fat dairy products. It also includes whole-grain products, fish, poultry and nuts. It is rich in potassium, magnesium and calcium as well as protein and fiber. It de-emphasizes, but does not eliminate, lean red meats, sweets, added sugars and sugar-containing beverages commonly found in the typical American diet. The DASH eating plan can be used for preventive measures as well as for people with specific dietary restrictions. It is not a vegetarian plan, and it does not require specialty foods.

For details about the DASH eating plan, and as a companion tool to use with this book, it is strongly recommended that you obtain a copy of *The DASH eating plan – Your Guide to Lowering your Blood Pressure with DASH*, (National Institute of Health, National Heart, Lung, and Blood Institute, revised April 2006.) It is downloadable at www.nhlbi.nih.gov/health/public/heart/hbp/dash/new_dash.pdf.

You can also order it online at www.nhlbi.nih.gov/ or call the NHLBI Health Information Center, 301-592-8573 or 240-629-3255.

Mailing address:
NHLBI Health Information Center
P.O. Box 30105
Bethesda, MD 20824-0105

Creativity is the key to using this book.

If you find counting calories stressful, then this book is written with you in mind. The recipes in this book are designed to help you stay within the goals of the DASH eating plan, as the nutrients, sodium, fat and cholesterol in each individual recipe are within range of the daily limit for each meal. The ingredients will give you ideas about

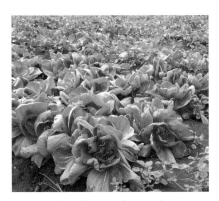

how to use locally-grown, farm-fresh produce, and locally-made products to bring excitement in your daily meals. Use the recipes as **guidelines**. They are not rigid formulas or magic bullets. Create variations by substituting similar ingredients for flavor, color or texture. For example, if the recipe calls for Shanghai cabbage, you can try substituting kale or *choy sum* (Chinese green-leaf cabbage). And salt, for instance, can be substituted with spices, vinegars and lemon zest. There is a wide variety of flavored vinegars for you to experiment with, and you can also try using different types of limes or citrus in place of lemon.

The DASH recommendations are a set of goals. As long as you maintain an average daily intake of the following values by weight (milligrams, or mg), over each day and each week, that is all you need to be concerned about. All this information is contained in most food labels. And the recipes in this book will give you ideas about the portion size that meet these goals.

DASH Daily Nutrient Goals	For a 2,100-calorie eating plan
% of Total Fat Calories	27%
% of Saturated Fat Calories	6%
Carbohydrate	55%
Cholesterol	150mg
Sodium	2,300mg*
Potassium	4,700mg
Calcium	1,250mg
Magnesium	500mg
Fiber	30g

According to the DASH eating plan, keeping a 1,500-mg daily goal for sodium is even more effective for lowering blood pressure among high-risk groups, including middle-aged and older individuals, African Americans, and those who have a genetic propensity for high blood pressure.

Lifestyle changes help prevent and control blood pressure.

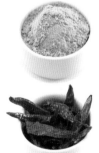

The two most important lifestyle elements that affect blood pressure and risk for getting heart disease are (1) eating habits, and (2) physical activities. To get the best results you have to combine a healthy eating plan with a regular physical activity program. A secondary, but equally important, result of these changes is weight control (or weight loss if you are overweight).

Doing things you like to do *and* eating well … how difficult is it for you to stay healthy?

Changing the type of foods you eat is only part of the strategy towards a healthier lifestyle. You have to think about what to do with the nutrients you ingest. The DASH eating plan calls for changes in **both** eating habits and physical activity. And if you find it difficult to stick to a consistent exercise regimen, as most people do, the DASH eating and activity plans are meant to help you. To start with, think about your favorite physical activities. Although there is some truth to "no pain, no gain," this book will help you "find treasure in your pleasure." You'll learn to focus on goals that are achievable within your weekly routine, and are enjoyable for you to do with significant others in your life. Once you get into a habit of doing regular physical activities that you really enjoy, you are on your way to a fun, sustainable and **healthy** lifestyle.

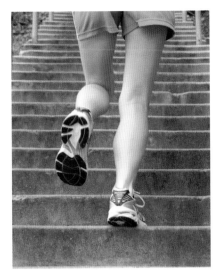

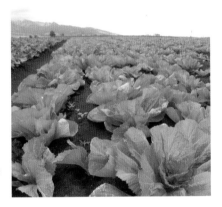

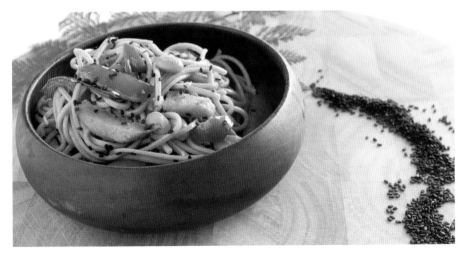

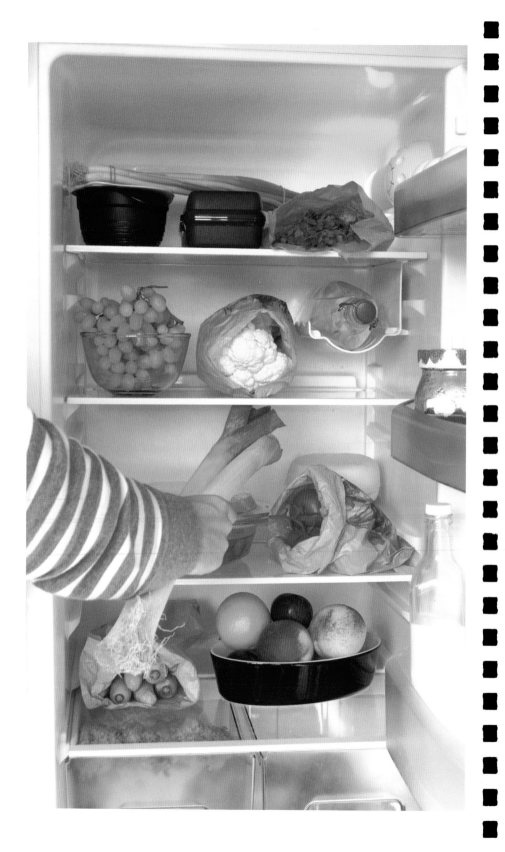

Chapter 2

A DASH of Nutrition

Grant Itomitsu
Registered Dietician, Instructor
Kapiʻolani Community College

You don't have to be a scientist to understand nutrition.

J ust yesterday, all the talk was about saturated fats, polyunsaturated and monounsaturated fats. Today it's the infamous trans fat or the highly-prized omega-3 fats with their EPA and DHA. Can someone pass me a microscope so I can cut out the trans-fatty acid from my piece of cake? We have effectively made eating into a great big complex scientific experiment. **Why can't we just KISS? "Keep It Simple ... Smarty-pants."**

All foods are meant to be eaten.

There is no such thing as good foods or bad foods. It is how we incorporate them into our lifestyle that leads to positive or negative consequences in health.

In all aspects of life, overindulgence or deficiency, there are consequences.

Remember, be sure to check with your physician and healthcare professional when changing your diet. People with certain health conditions may have slightly different nutritional needs. It is always best to speak with your healthcare provider to find out if you have specific nutritional needs.

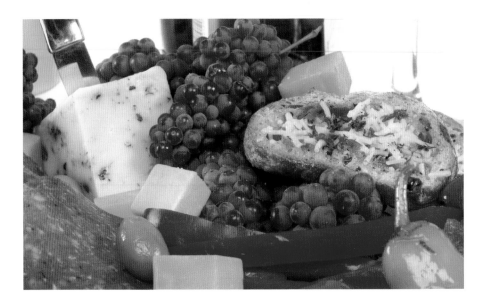

Balancing the "Ins" and "Outs"

Your entire life is based on balance. From your career and family to your finances and calories—balance is essential. In science we refer to this stability in the human body as "homeostasis." And when it refers to your diet, we hear a similar term, "moderation"—not too much and not too little—in essence a built-in set of scales. With food it comes down to a basic principle of energy in (the calories you put in your mouth) and energy out (the calories your body will burn with different activities).

Change Is Gradual

Stop looking for the easy way out. Think of eating as it truly is—a lifelong journey.

Unrealistic:
- Expect results to happen overnight.
- Rely on quick fixes for maintaining long-term health.
- Expect change with a lack of motivation and commitment.
- Make only short-term, temporary changes.

Realistic:
- Lose weight gradually. Losing just half a pound a week will result in a 26-pound weight loss in one year.
- Make small changes to your diet, not a complete overhaul. Think of one dietary habit you can change. Once you have ingrained your new habit, add another. Example: Cut out one bottle of soda or café mocha every day. Once it becomes habitual, then think of another area to improve upon.
- Don't think you have to eat perfectly at every single meal. Remember, eating is a lifelong journey. It is what you accomplish over a lifetime of eating, not just one meal. If you overindulge, balance out your intake for the rest of the day or week.

Think Before You Eat

Listen to your body; it will help you make better decisions. Learn how to identify your body's appetite. The following scale indicates the levels of hunger and satisfaction. Try to avoid the extremes on both ends of the spectrum as they relate to extreme hunger and overeating. Listen to your body's gentle cues that tell you when, and when not, to eat. It should not scream to you to "HURRY UP AND EAT NOW" (starving) or beg you to "STOP EATING BEFORE YOU BURST" (stuffed).

URGE TO SATISFACTION SCALE

Starving:	I could eat a horse. I need to eat, NOW!
Hungry:	My stomach is growling and mouth salivating. I am preoccupied with food.
Desire to eat:	I could use a bit to eat.
Satisfied:	I'm okay. Urge to eat has gone.
Full:	I had a little too much.
Stuffed:	Stick a fork in me, I'm done. Where's the sofa?

You can lose weight by eating ... here's how:

Motivation is the key. If you are motivated by food, this is the book for you. We want to motivate you to lose weight by eating fresh, flavorful and exciting food.

1. More variety, less boredom

- Limiting variety limits the amount of nutrients you get from foods. Aim to hit all the different food groups, such as grains, vegetables, fruits, dairy and meat.
- Most people lack vegetables and fruits in their diet. Find ways to incorporate them into your meals.
- Milk is not the only source of calcium. Try other dairy products such as cheese or yogurt (especially if you are lactose intolerant) or broccoli, most tofu and even sardines.
- Whole foods (fresh, unprocessed foods) are typically more nutrient dense than processed foods.

2. Focus on the foods you should eat more of in order to lose weight

- Figure out what food groups you're lacking, then gradually add food items that you enjoy to fill the voids. The new item will replace other food items that you are consuming in excess.
- Vegetables, whole grains and fruits are great to start with, as consumption is typically low.
- Select nutrient dense foods—foods that are low in calories yet filled with a lot of vitamins, minerals and fiber.
- Focus on fresh, whole foods, such as locally-grown produce, rather than highly-processed packaged foods.
- Foods are meant to be eaten, but not always in the quantities many

people consume. People often suffer from "portion distortion," an assumption that the portion they're eating is considered to be a healthy or normal amount. In most cases they grossly overestimate portion sizes. Be sure to read labels and familiarize yourself with proper portion sizes. (See page 43.)

*People with certain diseases may require a more thoughtful nutritional plan. Please check with your physician and healthcare provider.

3. Feed your body by balancing breakfast, lunch and dinner

- Think of your body as a car that needs fuel in order to run. At night, even while you sleep, your body utilizes calories. So in the morning you need to fuel up before you start your journey. That's why breakfast is truly the most important meal of the day. Not only does it provide you with the energy you need, but it also prevents feelings of extreme hunger throughout the day.

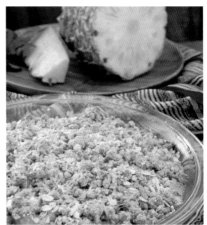

- If you skip breakfast, then by noon you will be "starving." (Remember what we discussed earlier about hunger levels.) People tend to overeat in order to compensate for their feeling of extreme hunger. Soon after a large lunch, you begin to feel a bit sleepy and become less productive. Then when you get home, you prepare a wonderful, well-meant dinner—a feast in many cases. After giving into gluttony, you put on your tennis shoes and run on the treadmill, mow the lawn, do some aerobics or take the dog for a five-mile walk, right? What? You don't do this? Then what is the

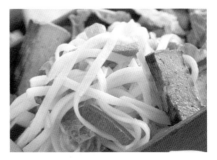

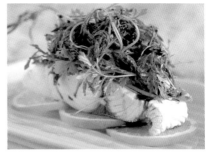

point of filling up with all that extra fuel? Okay, I get it … it's for energy for later use. Let me translate, "body fat." As with most people, you want to unwind from a hard day's work by reading the paper, watching TV or curling up with a good book. These activities do require energy, however they don't require as much energy as most people consume. Remember, energy in and energy out. Excess energy gets stored in your body as fat.

In general, we should rely on breakfast to provide us with the energy needed for the day. Have a light lunch. Then look at dinner as satiating your hunger, but not overwhelming it. Afterwards, a short, brisk 15-minute walk is ideal.

Easy Ways to Choose Good Food

1. Focus on Foods
Focus on food as a whole and don't get caught up with all the details. Leave the data to the scientists. The perfect food has not been discovered nor will it ever be. The human body is complex and requires variety. Feeding it, on the other hand, should be simple. So for now, treat your body well by feeding it properly, moving it consistently and giving it time to rest and recuperate. While diet is one part of the overall picture of optimal health, don't forget to exercise. (See the "A DASH to Action" chapter for suggestions on simple physical activities.)

A healthy diet is less overwhelming when you start with the three basics: fat, sugar and sodium.

Fats:
Fat comes in many different forms: saturated, trans, polyunsaturated, omega-3, cholesterol, monounsaturated, triglycerides. Instead of racking your brain with all the types of fats, keep it simple … smarty-pants (KISS) by following the tips below. With smart selections and good variety, the fat will take care of itself.

KISS: Focus on the foods rather than the fats.
- Select lean meats, which cuts back on the saturated fats, cholesterol, triglycerides.

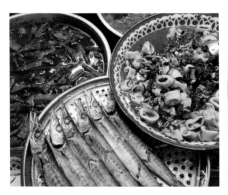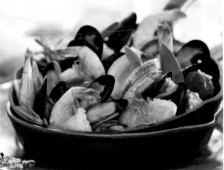

- Incorporate fish into the diet (getting some of the omega-3 fats). Now who wouldn't want to eat more *poke*? We have such a great abundance of Hawaiian seafood, why not take advantage of it?
- Use plant-based oils such as olive, canola, vegetable and flax seed oil instead of butter, palm oil, lard and tallow.
- Moderate how much oil you use. Using plant-based oils, such as olive oil, is not a carte blanche to use as much as you want.

Sugars:

Simple sugars come in many forms: Technical terms such as sucrose, glucose, fructose and dextrose are commonly used.

KISS: Decrease the amount of refined sugars.

- Look at food labels under the carbohydrate section and look for sugar. Practice common sense by moderating foods that have large concentrations in sugars, such as candies, cookies, sugary cereals, soda, juice drinks and pastries.

Sodium:

Sodium is found in many commonly used items. Use salt, *shoyu* (soy sauce), oyster sauce, *patis* (fish sauce) and *ajinomoto* (MSG) sparingly. Or use low-salt seasoning, such as lemon, spices and vinegar.

KISS: Control sodium intake when and where you can.

- Watch what you cannot control. Much of the sodium we take in comes from processed food as opposed to salt that is added during cooking or at the table. Sodium is added to foods for flavor and as a preservative. So canned foods, such as Vienna sausage, Spam, ham and even vegetables, have added sodium.

- Moderate the amount of sodium you use during cooking. Try not to add additional sodium at the table. Minimize use of processed food or look for low-sodium versions.

2. Whole vs. Processed, Farm vs. Factory
Select whole foods instead of processed foods, foods that are closer to the farm than the factory, and rely on natural foods for your nutrients rather than supplements.

KISS: Select whole, fresh foods over highly processed ones.
- Processed foods are often made from lower-quality ingredients, with added chemical flavoring agents to compensate for the inferior taste. Just take a look at the ingredients list and count how many chemicals you are eating.
- Farm-fresh, whole foods are packed with their natural flavors, plus many of the nutrients you need.
- Processed, factory-made foods often come with high level of sodium and sugar, which may contribute to health problems, such as high blood pressure and uncontrolled diabetes. These health problems over time may ultimately lead to more serious heart and kidney diseases.
- By making better food selections, using healthful cooking techniques and maintaining proper eating habits, you can reduce your health risks and save yourself a fortune on medical costs in the future.

How to Use Food Labels
Be sure to check the "serving size" and "servings per container" on food labels because the amount you typically consume may not reflect the serving size on the food label. You may assume that the food label is based on the consumption of the entire container, which may not be the case. Case in point: most people will consume an entire 20-ounce bottle of soda as a single serving. However, based on the food label, it is two and a half servings. Make sure to adjust the nutrients based on what you actually consume.

Food labels are based on a 2,000-calorie diet, which may not be the ideal amount for you. Nutrients that fall under the fat, carbohydrates and protein categories are based on the 2,000-calorie-a-day diet. Other nutrients such as sodium, potassium and cholesterol are based on set amounts, regardless of calories. In addition, the food label nutritional recommendations are not always the same as the DASH recommendations. However, they are typically in the same ballpark, with the exception of cholesterol.

The bottom line is that it's best to focus on the food label's "actual amounts" rather that the "percent daily values." This allows you to calculate nutrient amounts based on your own needs. You may want to keep a running total in your head of specific nutrients you need to focus on.

Remember, there is not a single perfect food, and sometimes food or meals will be outside of the DASH recommendations. Keep in mind, it's not about eating perfectly at each meal but rather how you balance your intake day to day, week to week, month to month and year to year for the rest of your life. Take enjoyment in the foods you eat while practicing moderation, variation and common sense.

Food labels are a quick and easy way to identify the nutrient content in foods. Check the actual amount (milligrams or mgs), not just the percent daily values. Compare the following below:

DASH Recommendations Versus Percent Daily Value

	DASH	FOOD LABELS
CALORIES	2,100kcals	2,000kcals
% of Calories from Fat	27%	30%
% of Calories from Saturated Fat	6%	10%
Cholesterol	150mg	300mg
Sodium	2,300mg	2,400mg
Fiber	30g	25g

Example: DASH eating plan sodium recommendation is 2,300mg while the Percent Daily Value* is based on 2,400mg. For cholesterol DASH is 150mg, not 300mg.

*Food labels list percentages that are based on recommended daily allowances—meaning the amount of nutrients a person should get each day. These numbers tell you the Percent Daily Value (DV) that one serving of this food provides as a percentage of established standards. For example, a label may show that a serving of the food provides 30 percent of the daily recommended amount of fiber. This means you still need another 70 percent to meet the recommended goal. Percent DV is based on a 2,000-calorie diet for adults older than 18. As a general rule of thumb, nutrition experts recommend limiting total fat, saturated fat, cholesterol and sodium in your diet, so choose foods with a lower Percent DV for these nutrients. Eat more foods with a higher Percent DV for vitamins, minerals and fiber.

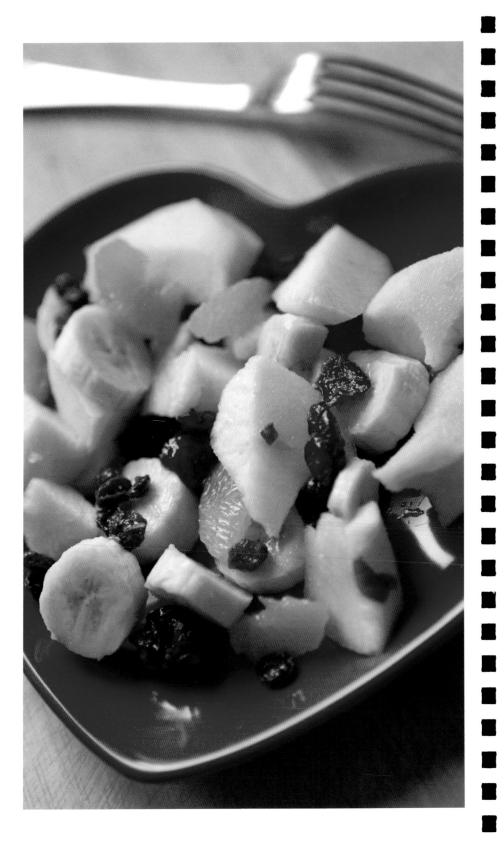

Chapter 3

The DASH Eating Plan
and Your Heart

The American Heart Association of Hawai'i

According to the National Institutes of Health (NIH) and the National Heart, Lung and Blood Institute (NHLBI), recent studies show that the combination of the DASH eating plan and a low sodium diet gives the biggest benefit for lowering blood pressure, or preventing the development of high blood pressure.

What Is Blood Pressure?

Two numbers are recorded when measuring your blood pressure, such as 117/78 mm Hg (millimeters of mercury). The top, or larger number (systolic pressure) measures the pressure in your arteries when your heart beats. The bottom, or smaller number (diastolic pressure) measures the pressure while your heart rests between beats.

What Is High Blood Pressure (for Adults 18 Years and Older)?

Blood Pressure Category	Systolic (mm Hg)		Diastolic (mm Hg)
Normal	Less than 120	and	Less than 80
Pre-hypertension	120-139	or	80-89
Hypertension, Stage 1	140-159	or	90-99
Hypertension, Stage 2	160 or higher	or	100 or higher

Source: Seventh Report of the Joint National Committee on Prevention, Detection, Evaluation and Treatment of High Blood Pressure (JNC 7 Complete Report) Hypertension 2003; 42:1206.

Hypertension is the medical term for high blood pressure. It doesn't refer to being tense, nervous or hyperactive. A person can be calm and relaxed and still have high blood pressure. High blood pressure usually has no symptoms. In 90 to 95 percent of high blood pressure cases, the cause is unknown. In the remaining 5 to 10 percent of cases, which are known as secondary hypertension, the causes could include kidney abnormality, a structural abnormality of the aorta existing since birth or narrowing of certain arteries. In fact, many people have high blood pressure for years without knowing it. That's why it's called the "silent killer." The only way to detect high blood pressure is to have a doctor or other qualified health professional check for it. It's a dangerous disease, not to be taken lightly!

Why Is High Blood Pressure Harmful?

High blood pressure causes the heart to work harder than normal. Both the heart and arteries are then more prone to injury. High blood pressure increases the risk of heart attacks, strokes, kidney failure, eye damage and congestive heart failure.

If high blood pressure is not treated, the heart may have to work harder to pump enough blood and oxygen to the body's organs and tissues. A heart forced to work harder than normal for a long time tends to enlarge and have a hard time doing its job.

High blood pressure also hurts arteries and arterioles (smaller arteries). Over time they become scarred, hardened and less elastic. This may occur as people age, but high blood pressure accelerates this process.

What Is Cholesterol?

Cholesterol is a soft, fat-like substance found in the bloodstream and in all of your body's cells. It's used to form cell membranes and some hormones, and is needed for other important functions. Cholesterol is part of a healthy body, but too much of it in your blood can be a problem. High blood cholesterol is a risk for heart disease and stroke. Cholesterol moves through your bloodstream to your body's cells in special carriers called

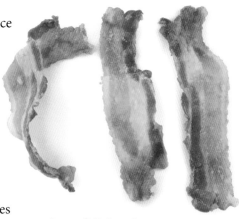

Source of LDL (bacon)

lipoproteins. There are many kinds of lipoproteins, but the two we most need to know about are low-density lipoprotein (LDL) and high-density lipoprotein (HDL). LDL cholesterol is "bad" cholesterol because it can build up in the inner walls of arteries through which blood travels to the heart and brain. Along with other substances, it forms plaque (a thick, hard, fatty deposit) that narrows the arteries and reduces blood flow. This condition is called atherosclerosis.

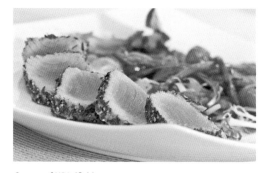

Source of HDL (fish)

HDL cholesterol is "good" cholesterol because it seems to lower your risk of heart attack and stroke. Medical experts believe HDL carries cholesterol away from the arteries and back to the liver, where it's passed from the body.

What Do Cholesterol Numbers Mean?

Total Cholesterol Level	Category
Less than 200 mg/dL	Desirable
200–239 mg/dL	Borderline High
240 mg/dL and above	High Blood Cholesterol

What Can Be Done About High Blood Pressure and High Blood Cholesterol?

Dietary and lifestyle changes help control high blood pressure and high blood cholesterol. A healthy diet and lifestyle are the best weapons you have to fight cardiovascular disease. It's not as hard as you may think! Remember, it is the overall pattern of choices you make that counts.

- The American Heart Association/American Stroke Association advises people to **eat lots of fruits and vegetables, and to eat fat-free and low-fat dairy products**. Such diets are rich in potassium, calcium, magnesium and protein, and low in saturated fat, total fat and cholesterol. These foods are nutrient rich and lower in calories, and can help you control your weight and blood pressure.
- The American Heart Association/American Stroke Association recommends that you **limit your intake of saturated fats** to less than 7 percent of total daily calories, and less than 1 percent for trans fats. Your body makes some cholesterol. The food you eat is responsible for the rest. Commonly eaten cholesterol-containing foods include whole milk, eggs, shellfish and organ meats such as liver.

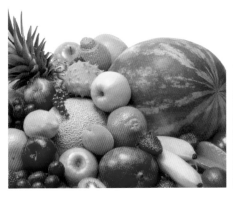
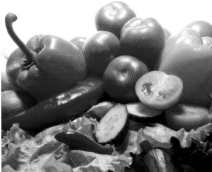

- Some people can lower their blood pressure by reducing **sodium** (salt) in their diet. This means avoiding salty foods and cutting down on salt in cooking and at the table.
- Drinking too much **alcohol** (more than one ounce of pure alcohol, or two drinks per day for men and one drink per day for women) raises blood pressure in some people and should be restricted. Alcoholic drinks are high in non-nutritious calories, and may cause weight gain.
- Many people who have high blood pressure are **overweight or obese**. Obesity is a risk factor for both high blood pressure and heart disease. When people lose weight, their blood pressure often drops, too.
- Regular **physical activity** helps control weight and lower blood pressure. Being active brings many benefits for your heart and your health. How much activity do you need? Aim to get at least 30 minutes of moderate physical activity on most, if not all, days of the week. If you are trying to lose weight, aim for 30 to 60 minutes on most days.
- For some people, losing weight, reducing sodium and other lifestyle changes won't lower high blood pressure and/or high blood cholesterol as much as needed. Those people will probably need to take **medication** and should consult a healthcare provider.

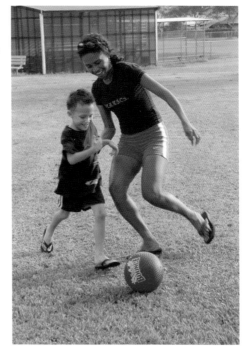

Make exercise a part of your daily life.

Are You at Risk for a Heart Attack or Stroke?

If you check two or more boxes, see a healthcare provider for a complete assessment of your risks!

❑ **AGE AND GENDER:** I am a man over 45 years old; OR I am a woman over 55 years old.

❑ **FAMILY HISTORY:** My father or brother had a heart attack before age 55; OR my mother or sister had one before age 65; OR my mother, father, sister, brother or grandparent had a stroke.

❑ **HEART DISEASE MEDICAL HISTORY:** I have a coronary heart disease, atrial fibrillation or another heart condition(s); OR I've had a heart attack.

❑ **STROKE MEDICAL HISTORY:** I've been told that I have carotid artery disease; OR I've had a stroke or TIA (transient ischemic attack); OR I have a disease of the leg arteries, a high red blood cell count or sickle cell anemia.

❑ **BLOOD PRESSURE:** My blood pressure is 140/90 mm Hg or higher; OR a health professional has said my blood pressure is too high; OR I don't know what my blood pressure is.

❑ **TOBACCO SMOKE:** I smoke; OR I'm exposed to other people's smoke regularly.

❑ **TOTAL CHOLESTEROL:** My total cholesterol is 240 mg/dL or higher; OR I don't know my level.

❑ **HDL CHOLESTEROL:** My HDL ("good") cholesterol is less than 40 mg/dL; OR I don't know my HDL cholesterol level.

❑ **PHYSICAL ACTIVITY:** I get less than a total of 30 minutes of physical activity on most days.

❑ **OVERWEIGHT:** I am at least 20 pounds overweight for my body-type.

❑ **DIABETES:** I have diabetes (a fasting blood sugar of 126 mg/dL or higher); OR I need medicine to control my blood sugar. 🫐

Chapter 4

The DASH Eating Plan and Your Kidneys

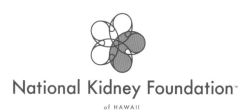

National Kidney Foundation™
of HAWAII

- One in nine American adults are affected by Chronic Kidney Disease (CKD) and in Hawai'i the statistic is closer to one in seven.
- Many of Hawai'i's ethnic groups are at higher risk, including Filipinos, Native Hawaiians and Japanese.
- Individuals with CKD often have no symptoms until 70 percent of kidney function is lost, and you cannot get it back.
- **Diabetes and high blood pressure (hypertension)** are the two leading causes of Chronic Kidney Disease.
- CKD progression can be slowed or prevented if it is detected in the early stages and managed with diet, exercise and medications.
- Once you have reached the stage of kidney failure, the only remaining life-saving options are long-term dialysis or a kidney transplant.

You are at higher risk for chronic diseases such as kidney disease, diabetes and/or high blood pressure if:

- You don't get much physical activity.
- You have unhealthy eating habits.
- You are overweight.
- You have family members (blood relatives) with kidney disease, diabetes and/or high blood pressure.
- You are of Asian, Pacific Islander or African-American ancestry.

The two most important steps you can take:

1. Eat healthier and increase physical activity.
2. Maintain good control of blood pressure and diabetes.

Diabetes and Your Kidneys

Diabetes is the leading cause of kidney disease and is a serious health problem that occurs when your body has **too much sugar (glucose) in the blood**. Sugar is needed for fuel, but when there is too much for the body to handle, it can cause big problems for your kidneys, eyes, nerves, heart and other parts of your body. Some people get diabetes young and that is called Type 1, or juvenile onset. You can also get it as an adult and that is Type 2, or adult onset diabetes. The main risk factors for Type 2 diabetes are being overweight, lack of physical activity and a poor diet. **It is essential to keep blood sugar levels within the normal limits of 70-110.** Diabetes that is not well controlled damages the small blood vessels of the body. That is why diabetics have foot and eye problems. Poorly controlled diabetes can also cause high blood pressure, hardening of the arteries, urinary tract infections, damage to nerves that control the bladder and kidney damage.

Diet, High Blood Pressure and Your Kidneys

High blood pressure, or hypertension, is the second leading cause of kidney disease. Pressure moves the blood from the heart to other organs. With hypertension, the increased high force of your blood pushes against the walls of your arteries, causing damage that keeps kidneys from functioning properly. Individuals with a family history of high blood pressure or who are overweight, eat a diet high in sodium and/or smoke, are at increased risk for high blood pressure. It is recommended that your blood pressure be maintained at 120/80. Keeping blood pressure under control with a proper diet, physical activity, weight reduction, stopping smoking and taking prescribed medication will help to protect your kidneys from irreversible damage.

Some signs and symptoms of chronic kidney disease:

According to the National Kidney Foundation, the following are possible signs and symptoms of kidney disease:

- high blood pressure
- blood or protein in the urine
- difficult, painful or more frequent urination, especially at night
- puffiness around the eyes, and swelling of the hands and feet
- fatigue or lack of energy
- nausea and vomiting, poor appetite, hiccups, weight loss
- trouble sleeping, itching, leg cramping at night and trouble breathing

> For more detailed information or testing for signs and symptoms of chronic kidney disease, contact the National Kidney Foundation of Hawai'i for more information.
>
> **1314 S. King St., Suite #305
> Honolulu, HI 96814
> 808-593-1515 or
> 1-800-488-2277
> www.kidneyhi.org**

Please be sure to check with your physician if you feel that you may have one or more of these symptoms. Chronic kidney disease often has no symptoms until the disease is quite advanced—this is why it is called "the silent killer."

How do I prevent and/or slow kidney disease?

- Control and/or avoid developing high blood pressure.
- Lower your LDL cholesterol ("bad" cholesterol) if it is higher than 100.
- Make healthy food choices.
- Engage in regular physical activity.
- Quit smoking.
- Limit alcohol use.
- Manage and/or prevent diabetes.

Eating a balanced diet is an important part of good health for everyone, not just people with CKD.

The DASH eating plan helps you stay healthy with these key ingredients:

Protein

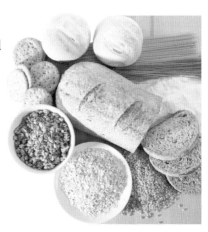

- The main sources are meats, poultry, cheese, milk, eggs, fish, plus some vegetables like peas and beans.
- Helps your body to grow, replace tissue, make hormones, enzymes and antibodies.
- The kidneys break down the waste product of protein digestion, called urea.
- Eat smaller portions of protein more often.
- Get adequate protein by concentrating on high-quality protein, and add herbs and spices to enhance flavor.
- High-protein diets are not advised for people with chronic kidney disease, especially not those on dialysis.

Carbohydrates

- The main sources are grains, fruits and starchy vegetables.
- Major source of energy and helps body use other nutrients.
- Not eating enough carbohydrates may cause you to feel tired or lose weight.
- Supply energy and other important nutrients like B vitamins, fiber, iron and potassium.

Fats

- We need to eat some fat to help our bodies function well, but the typical person usually eats too much fat.
- Important source of energy; has twice the calories of protein and carbohydrates.
- Provides essential fatty acids for growth and functioning.

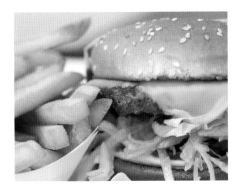

- **Two types:**
  o Saturated fat: solid at room temperature (butter, coconut oil, lard, cocoa butter, palm oil)
  o Unsaturated fat: liquid vegetable oils (olive, canola, safflower, corn, soybean, sunflower seed)
- A high-fat diet can raise cholesterol and triglyceride levels in the blood. These fatty substances can build up in your blood vessels and over time can block them off, causing heart disease and high blood pressure that will damage your kidneys.
- High fat intake is also linked to diabetes and some forms of cancer. And as we discussed, diabetes is the leading cause of chronic kidney disease.

What foods are high in fat?

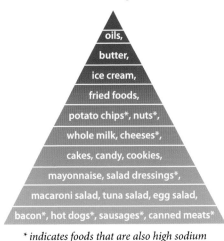

oils,
butter,
ice cream,
fried foods,
potato chips*, nuts*,
whole milk, cheeses*,
cakes, candy, cookies,
mayonnaise, salad dressings*,
macaroni salad, tuna salad, egg salad,
bacon*, hot dogs*, sausages*, canned meats*

indicates foods that are also high sodium

- **Here are a few suggestions for cutting back on the fat:**
  - Avoid fried foods. Eat fewer high-fat foods.
  - Use a non-stick pot or pan. Use non-stick spray instead of butter, margarine or oil.
  - Read food labels to look for hidden fat.
  - Trim all the excess fat off of meat and remove skin from chicken and turkey.
  - Reduce meat consumption and prepare extra vegetables as a substitute.

Potassium

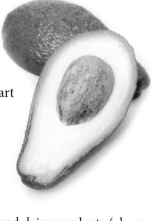

- Mineral found in many foods, especially fruits and vegetables.
- Keeps nerves and muscles working properly.
- Poorly managed potassium levels can cause heart problems.
- The main sources of potassium are potatoes, bananas, tomatoes, avocados, prunes, raisins and other dried fruits, cantaloupe and honeydew melons, oranges and tangerines, dried beans and peas, nuts and seeds, dark-green and leafy vegetables such as spinach, and milk and dairy products (cheese, yogurt, ice cream, etc.) and salt substitutes.
- For people who need to reduce the amount of potassium in their food as recommended by their physicians, you can "leach" your vegetables before you cook or eat them. Peel and cut the vegetable thinly, soak in water for several hours, discard the water and prepare the vegetables. Drain all liquids from canned vegetables or fruits before use.
- The DASH eating plan can be high in potassium.

Sodium

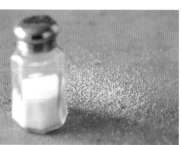

- Mineral that helps regulate fluid content in the body.
- You need sodium in your body to help control blood pressure, but high sodium intake can lead to high blood pressure and cause damage to your kidneys.
- Too much sodium can make you thirsty and cause fluid overload, shortness of breath and high blood pressure.
- The main sources are table salt, foods eaten out and take-out foods, processed and luncheon meats, most canned and frozen foods, condiments such as catsup and mustard, salty seasonings and soy sauce, chips and pickles.
- How to use less sodium:
  - o Use herbs and spices instead of salt.
  - o Buy fresh rather than processed foods.
  - o Avoid using large quantity of salty condiments, such as soy sauce, oyster sauce, fish sauces like *patis* (Philippine fish sauce), and *nuoc*

mam (Vietnamese), *bagoong* (Philippine fish paste), *harm ha* (Chinese shrimp paste), relish, pickles, mustard, etc.

o Use low-sodium version of condiments, such as low-sodium soy sauce, and natural flavor enhancers and seasonings (lemon juice, vinegar, citrus and spices).

You should know, though, that there is no such thing as a "one-size-fits-all" diet.

1. Each diet plan will be customized to your individual needs depending on your health status.
2. People differ in many ways: medically, physically and culturally.
3. Some people with chronic kidney disease may need to limit their intakes of protein, phosphorus, sodium and potassium. Tailoring your diet can make a big difference both in the early stages of chronic kidney disease and with kidney failure.
4. The DASH eating plan is high in potassium and phosphorus, and the amounts of protein may be more than a person with CKD should eat. Consult a Registered Dietitian or physician to learn which diet changes are right for you.

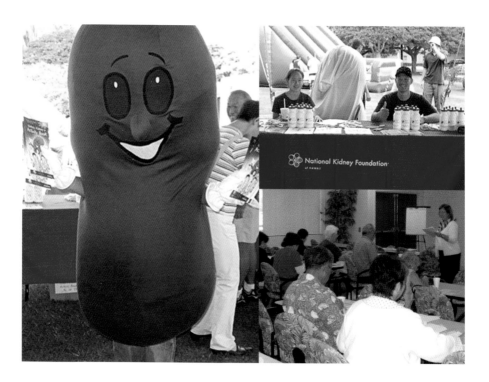

The National Kidney Foundation of Hawai'i recommends the **right foods** in the **right amount** at the **right time**.

Eating the RIGHT FOODS means:

Vegetables:
Salad greens, broccoli, tomatoes, carrots, etc. Vegetables are naturally low in fat and you can fill your stomach with these tasty foods! Season with low-fat salad dressings, herbs/spices or small amounts of flavored oils.

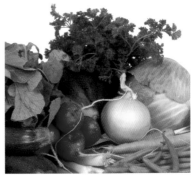

Breads, grains/cereals (starches):
Rice, noodles, poi, breads, cereals and crackers, etc. These foods provide the main fuel for the body. Read food labels for hidden fat or cholesterol, and pay attention to portion control.

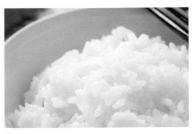

Proteins (Meats):
Meat, fish, poultry, eggs, beans, nuts/seeds, tofu/soy products (meat substitutes). Most people only need 5 to 7 ounces from the protein foods group A DAY.

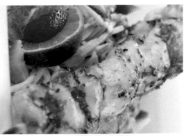

Fruit:
Fruits include bananas, papayas, apples, watermelon, cantaloupe, strawberries, etc. Fruits are "nature's candy" and can provide a sweet and healthy treat. Just beware of how much you eat at one time.

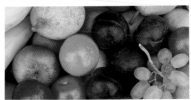

Dairy group:
Foods in this group include milk, yogurt cheese and cottage cheese. Foods from this group are a good source of calcium. Choose fat-free (skim) or low-fat (1 percent) milk or yogurt, to cut down on your fat intake.

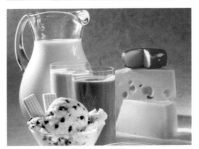

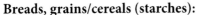

Eating the RIGHT AMOUNT means:

- 1/2 of your plate is for vegetables (containing potassium).
- 1/4 of your plate is for the breads/grains/cereals group.
- 1/4 of your plate for meat (containing protein and phosphorous).
- Add 1 serving of fruit next to your plate (containing potassium).
- Add 1 serving (8 ounces) from the dairy group (containing protein and phosphorous).

Portion control is important!

* You can create your own reference measurements in other ways that are convenient and easy to remember.

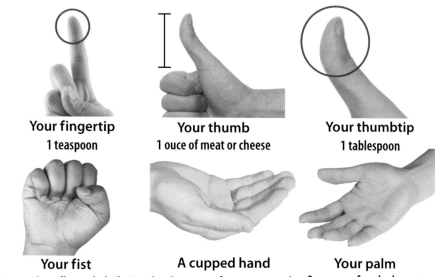

Your fingertip
1 teaspoon

Your thumb
1 ouce of meat or cheese

Your thumbtip
1 tablespoon

Your fist
1 cup or 1 medium whole fruit

A cupped hand
1 to 2 ounces of nuts or pretzels

Your palm
3 ounces of cooked meat, poultry or fish

Look for the "Nutrition Facts" on food labels to learn:

- How much is in one serving
- How much fat is in one serving
- How many calories are in that serving
- How many total servings are in the container
- The nutritional value per serving

Some tips to help you if you need them:

1. **Less sodium:** Look for foods labeled no added salt, low sodium, very low sodium, or unsalted and use spices and herbs.
2. **Less added sugar:** Look for foods labeled no sugar, packed in juice or light/lite syrup, 100-percent juice, sugar-free (if you have diabetes, read labels for carbohydrates).
3. **Less fat:** Look for foods labeled fat-free, low-fat, less-fat, reduced-fat, light or lite, lean, extra lean.
4. **Less milk/dairy:** Use non-dairy substitutes.

Eating at the RIGHT TIME means:

- Eat three regularly spaced meals per day.
- Avoid skipping meals.
- Eat your meals at about the same time each day.

Eating at regular times is like making sure that your gas tank is properly filled. If you skip a refill (a meal), you might run out of gas (energy). On the other hand, eating very large amounts of food only once or twice a day is like trying to overfill your gas tank. The excess that cannot be used is stored as fat! That's why it is important to eat regular meals.

Now that we've talked about healthier eating, let's talk about physical activity.

Being physically active has lots of benefits for your kidneys!

Being active can:

Lower blood sugar
Lower blood pressure
Lower your cholesterol
Make your heart and bones stronger
Give you more energy throughout the day
Help you lose weight or prevent weight gain
Help you to sleep better
Relieve stress

Are you physically active?

NKFH disclaimer:

The DASH and DASH-Low Sodium diets were tested on people with blood pressures less than 160/80-95, who did not have medical problems, such as poorly controlled diabetes, hyperlipidemia, and recent heart attacks, who were not taking medications for their blood pressures. These diets are widely recommended for the treatment and prevention of hypertension because the studies were very well-designed, the diets were prepared for the participants and the studies were large enough to yield statistically significant results. Because of the cost and complexity, these studies have not been replicated in people with other medical conditions.

People with chronic kidney disease frequently have other medical problems, may be on medications, and have other dietary restrictions. While many of the recipes in this book are tasty and suitable, people with CKD may wish to check with their Registered Dietitian, physician or other knowledgeable health care professional before following the DASH eating plan.

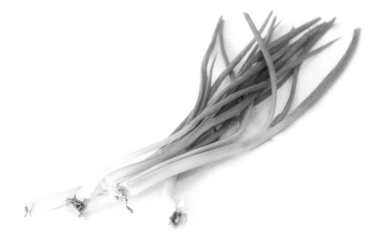

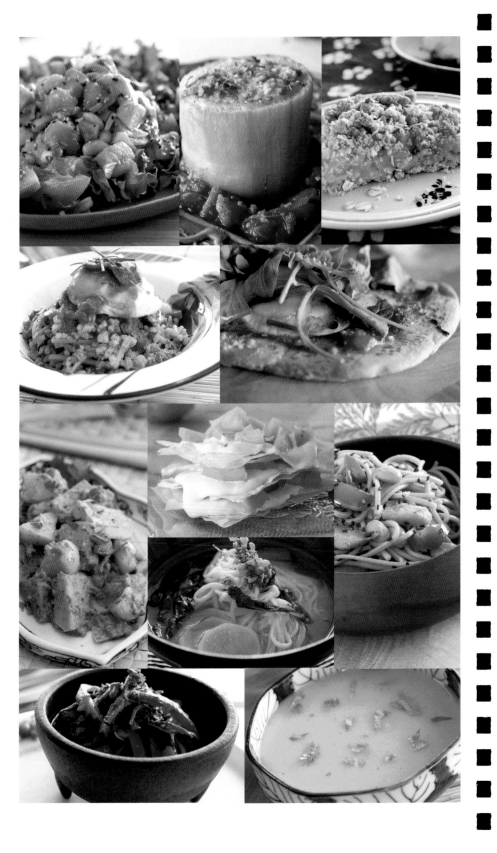

Chapter 5

70 <u>DASH Recipes</u>

Banana Gingerbread

By: Alyssa Moreau

6 servings

Whole-wheat pastry flour	1 1/2 cups	Rice, soy, almond or low-fat milk	2/3 cup
Wheat germ, toasted	1/4 cup	Macadamia nut oil	2 tbsp.
Baking powder	1 1/2 tsp.	Ginger, fresh, pressed to extract juice*	2" piece
Baking soda	1/4 tsp.	Molasses	2 tbsp.
Egg, or 1tbsp. of egg replacer		Hawaiian lehua honey	2 tbsp.
(Ener-G or BiPro)	1 each	Ginger, crystallized, chopped fine	1 tbsp.
Ginger, ground	1 tsp.	Golden raisins (optional)	1 to 2 tbsp.
Cinnamon	1 tsp.		
Banana, mashed-ripe, Apple			
or Williams	1 cup		

1. Combine the dry ingredients together and mix well.
2. Blend together the banana, rice milk, oil, fresh ginger, molasses and honey.
3. Add banana mixture to the dry ingredients, with the crystallized ginger and raisins.
4. Stir until the dry ingredients are moistened, then pour batter into an oiled 9" pie plate or 8"x8" baking pan.
5. Bake at 350 degrees for 20 to 25 minutes.

* Press peeled ginger through a garlic press to extract juice; strain through a fine mesh strainer.

A wholesome breakfast bread, light on excess sweeteners and unhealthy oils and egg-free, this can be baked ahead of time, sliced and stored in the freezer for enjoyment at a later date. You can also make into muffins (bake at 350 degrees for about 17 minutes; check with a toothpick) and take to work or a carry as a snack.

Whole-wheat pastry flour, wheat germ and dry egg replacer are standard items at local health food stores. Don't hesitate to venture in and browse around. If you cannot find it on the shelves, ask a store employee for help.

Nutrition Facts	
Serving Size (126g)	
Amount Per Serving	
Calories 310	Calories from Fat 60
	% Daily Value*
Total Fat 7g	11%
Saturated Fat 0.5g	3%
Trans Fat 0g	
Cholesterol 0mg	0%
Sodium 230mg	10%
Total Carbohydrate 54g	18%
Dietary Fiber 7g	28%
Sugars 17g	
Protein 9g	

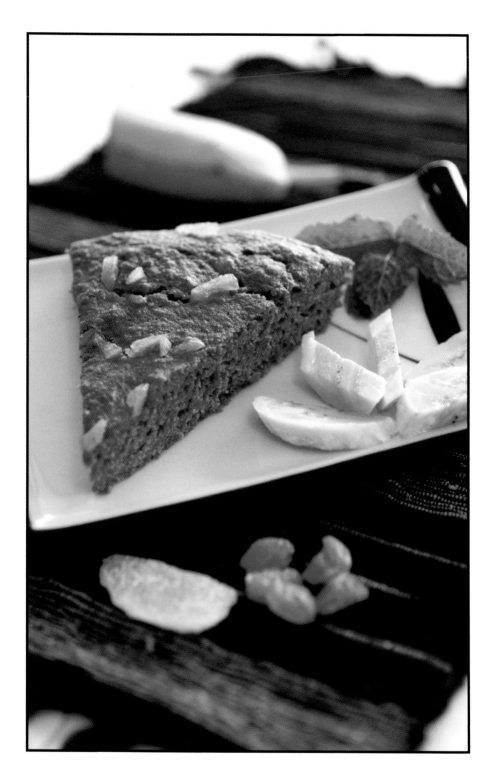

Breakfast Naan/Pizza with Arugula

By: Sharon Kobayashi

4 servings

Naan* or whole-wheat pita bread, low-salt	4 each
Marinara sauce	1/4 cup
Parmesan cheese, freshly grated	4 tbsp. (1 oz.)
Eggs	4 each
Arugula, finely sliced	1 cup (1 oz.)

*Naan is an Indian flat bread. The Indialife brand has less salt and fat than many other forms of flat bread. It can be substituted with any low/no-salt corn tortilla or flat bread.

1. Pre-heat oven to 400 degrees.
2. Spray each flat bread on one side with cooking spray.
3. Lay flat bread (spray side down) on baking sheet.
4. Top each with 1 tbsp. of marinara sauce, spread to thin layer.
5. Sprinkle 1 tbsp. of cheese and crack an egg onto each flatbread.
6. Bake for about 12 to 15 minutes, or until egg is set.
7. Place each pizza on a plate. Sprinkle each with 1/4 cup arugula.
8. Serve immediately.

For easy, fresh grated Parmesan, dice a small quantity at a time (3 to 4 oz.) from the block. Pulse in food processor until grated consistency. Keep in a tightly covered container in the refrigerator.

Nutrition note: This recipe uses a whole egg for each person, which raises the cholesterol level per serving in the nutrition label for this recipe. The DASH dietary approach is about balancing intake over a period of time. Unless you are under specific dietary restrictions, and as long as you reduce the cholesterol intake from other food during the same period, the DASH eating plan allows for an egg intake of no more than four per week.

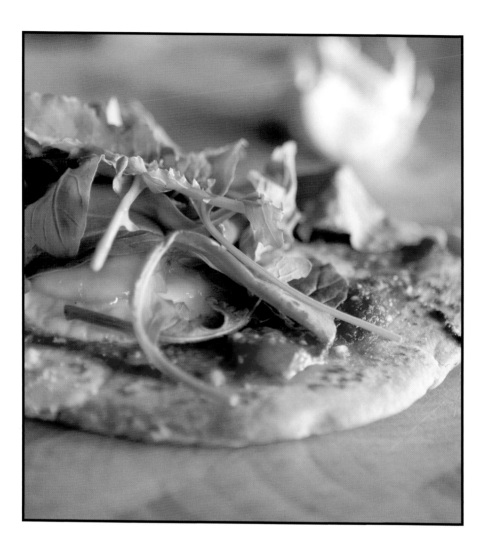

Nutrition Facts

Serving Size (120g)

Amount Per Serving

Calories 260   Calories from Fat 100

	% Daily Value*
Total Fat 11g	**17**%
Saturated Fat 2.5g	**13**%
Trans Fat 0g	
Cholesterol 190mg	**63**%
Sodium 420mg	**18**%
Total Carbohydrate 26g	**9**%
Dietary Fiber 2g	**8**%
Sugars 2g	
Protein 13g	

6 servings

Dried fruit of choice (pineapple, dried apple, mango, apricot)	1/2 cup
Whole-wheat pastry flour	1 cup
Oat flour	1/2 cup
Baking powder	2 tsp.
Egg replacer (BiPro or Ener-G)	1 tbsp.
Agave syrup* (maple may also be substituted)	1/3 cup
Ginger, powder	1 tsp.
Ginger, fresh, grated (optional)	1 tsp.
Cinnamon	1 tsp.
Salt	1/4 tsp.
Bran	3/4 cup
Soy milk, unsweetened Silk or Vitasoy or low-fat milk	1 1/4 cups
Light oil (high-oleic safflower or organic canola)	3 tbsp.
Applesauce	3 tbsp.
Vanilla	1 tsp.
Maple flavor (optional)	1/2 tsp.
Ginger, crystallized, chopped	1/4 cup

1. Preheat oven to 350 degrees.
2. Lightly oil a 9" pie plate.
3. Combine dry ingredients in a mixing bowl. Separately, combine the wet ingredients and then add to the dry mix.
4. Add the crystallized ginger and stir until just combined.
5. Pour into prepared pie plate and bake for 10 to 12 minutes or until a toothpick inserted in the center comes out clean. Alternatively, you can pour the batter into muffin tins; bake for 12 to 15 minutes.

* Agave syrup is available at the local health food stores and has a very low glycemic index level.

Nutrition Facts

Serving Size (151g)

Amount Per Serving

Calories 360	Calories from Fat 90

% Daily Value*

Total Fat 10g	**15%**
Saturated Fat 1g	**5%**
Trans Fat 0g	
Cholesterol 0mg	**0%**
Sodium 330mg	**14%**
Total Carbohydrate 66g	**22%**
Dietary Fiber 7g	**28%**
Sugars 24g	
Protein 8g	

Poha Jelly "Puddle" Scones

By: Alyssa Moreau

4 servings

Flour	1 cup
Whole-wheat flour	1/3 cup
Salt	1/4 tsp.
Baking powder	1/2 tsp.
Sugar	1 tbsp.
Oil	3 tbsp.
Milk, low-fat	1/2 cup
Vinegar	1 tsp.
Jelly or jam, Poha or guava, mango, strawberry-guava or liliko'i	4 tbsp.

1. Preheat oven to 375 degrees.
2. Mix first 5 ingredients together in a mixing bowl.
3. Separately, stir together the oil, milk and vinegar. Add to the dry mixture and stir with a spoon until a ball forms.
4. Put on a floured board and knead 8 to 10 times.
5. Cut into four equal parts. Shape into rounds about 3/4" thick.
6. With the back of a spoon, make an indentation in the middle of each scone. Fill indentation with favorite Hawaiian jelly or jam.
7. Place on a non-stick pan and bake for approximately 12 to 15 minutes.

Options: Jelly/Jam can be omitted and dried fruit such as mango, banana, papaya, pineapple, can be added to the dough. For larger scones, divide dough into three parts.

Dough can be shaped into a large round and then cut into pie-shaped pieces.

Nutrition Facts

Serving Size (105g)

Amount Per Serving

Calories 310   Calories from Fat 100

	% Daily Value*
Total Fat 11g	**17%**
Saturated Fat 1g	**5%**
Trans Fat 0g	
Cholesterol 0mg	**0%**
Sodium 230mg	**10%**
Total Carbohydrate 47g	**16%**
Dietary Fiber 2g	**8%**
Sugars 18g	
Protein 5g	

Passion Fruit Pain De Perdu with Seasonal Fruit and Cheesecake Cream
By: Sharon Kobayashi

2 servings

Strawberries, mango or other soft, seasonal fruit, diced	1 cup
Banana, sliced	1 each
Passion fruit, pulp and juice only	1 each (about 2 tbsp.)
Sugar	2 tbsp.
Egg whites (or 1/2 cup Egg Beaters)	4 each
Orange juice	1/4 cup
Vanilla extract	1 tsp.
Whole-grain bread	4 slices
Butter, unsalted	1 tsp.
Cheesecake cream (see recipe below)	6 tbsp.

1. Combine fruit with passion fruit and sugar and macerate for at least 10 minutes.
2. Combine eggs, orange juice and vanilla, and then whisk until incorporated.
3. Quickly dredge 1 slice of bread in egg mixture, transfer to a plate and top with 3 tbsp. of cheese cake cream.
4. Quickly dredge another slice of bread and top sandwich. Repeat.
5. Cover sandwiches and refrigerate at least 10 minutes.
6. In a large skillet, melt 1 tsp. butter on medium heat, add sandwiches and cook until golden brown.
7. Add remaining tsp. of butter, flip sandwiches and cook until golden brown.
8. To serve, top each sandwich with half of the macerated fruit, drizzling the fruit syrup over.

Tip: Make cheesecake cream the night before.

Cheesecake Cream
2 servings

Ricotta cheese, low-fat	1/2 cup
Lemon zest (or lemon extract)	1/4 tsp.
Vanilla extract	1/2 tsp.
Powdered sugar	2 tbsp.

1. Add all ingredients into food processor.
2. Blend until very smooth and creamy, scrapping down sides as needed.
3. Store covered, in refrigerator. Best to let rest overnight before using.

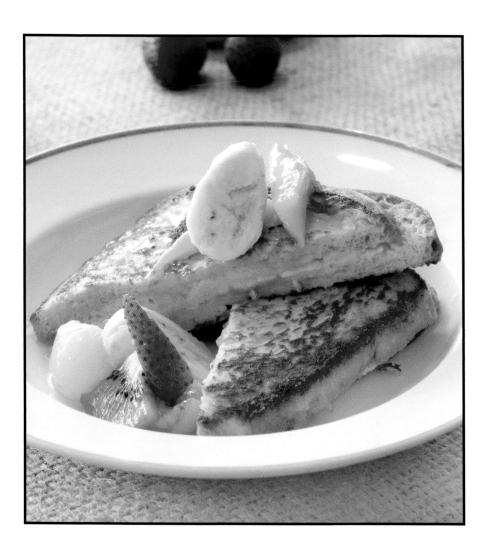

Nutrition Facts

Serving Size (402g)

Amount Per Serving

Calories 430   Calories from Fat 50

% Daily Value*

Total Fat 6g	**9%**
Saturated Fat 3g	**15%**
Trans Fat 0g	
Cholesterol 20mg	**7%**
Sodium 330mg	**14%**
Total Carbohydrate 83g	**28%**
Dietary Fiber 14g	**56%**
Sugars 46g	
Protein 18g	

6 servings

Rolled oats	4 cups	Apple juice	1/4 cup
Wheat germ	1/2 cup	Almond extract	1 tsp.
Cinnamon	1 tsp.	Assorted dried fruits: pineapple,	
Salt	1/4 tsp.	mango, papaya, banana	1 cup
Macadamia nut oil	2 tbsp.	Unsweetened coconut, shredded	1/8 cup
Hawaiian lehua honey	1/4 cup		

1. In a large bowl, mix together the oats, wheat germ, cinnamon and salt.
2. In a liquid measuring cup, combine the liquid ingredients and stir well.
3. Pour over oat mixture and toss to coat everything evenly.
4. Spread in an even layer on a cookie sheet.
5. Bake at 325 degrees for 15 minutes.
6. Reduce heat to 185 degrees and bake for 10 to 15 minutes more or until nicely brown and crisp.
7. Mix in the dried fruit and coconut.
8. Cool and store in an airtight container.

Serving suggestion: Good with plain, non-fat yogurt and fresh fruit or as a cereal with soy, almond or non-fat milk.

Nutrition Facts

Serving Size (117g)

Amount Per Serving

Calories 430　　　Calories from Fat 90

	% Daily Value*
Total Fat 10g	**15**%
Saturated Fat 1g	**5**%
Trans Fat 0g	
Cholesterol 0mg	**0**%
Sodium 150mg	**6**%
Total Carbohydrate 73g	**24**%
Dietary Fiber 9g	**36**%
Sugars 32g	
Protein 12g	

Makes 12 muffins

Whole-wheat pastry flour	2 cups	Unsweetened apple juice	
Baking powder	2 tsp.	concentrate	3/4 cup
Baking soda	1/2 tsp.	Rice, soy or other low-fat milk	1/2 cup
Egg replacer (equivalent to 2 eggs)	2 tbsp.	Macadamia nut oil	1 tbsp.
Water	4 tbsp.	Hawaiian lehua honey	6 tbsp.
Macadamia or other nut butter			
(i.e., almond, peanut or cashew)	3/4 cup		

(Recipe continues on next page.)

1. Preheat oven to 350 degrees.
2. Mix flour, baking powder and baking soda together in a medium bowl.
3. In another bowl, mix the egg replacer with water, and then add nut butter until smooth.
4. Mix in apple juice concentrate, rice milk and oil; beat until well blended.
5. Add the nut butter mixture to the dry ingredients. Stir until just mixed.
6. Fill paper-lined muffin tins 1/2 full with batter. Make a small indentation in the batter with a spoon and place 1/2 tbsp. honey in each center.
7. Top with remaining batter to cover.
8. Bake until top springs back lightly when pressed, approximately 25 minutes.
9. Cool 5 minutes on rack before serving.

Nutrition Facts

Serving Size (73g)

Amount Per Serving

Calories 240 Calories from Fat 120

	% Daily Value*
Total Fat 13g	20%
Saturated Fat 7g	35%
Trans Fat 0g	
Cholesterol 30mg	10%
Sodium 150mg	6%
Total Carbohydrate 29g	10%
Dietary Fiber 3g	12%
Sugars 12g	
Protein 3g	

Hawaiian-Style Oatmeal

By: Alyssa Moreau

2 to 3 servings

Water, boiling	1 1/2 cups	Salt	1/4 tsp.
Milk, low-fat, or rice, soy or almond milk	1 1/2 cups	Cinnamon	1 tsp.
Oats	1 cup	Maple syrup	2 tbsp.
Ginger, crystallized, chopped	1 tbsp.	Banana, sliced	1 cup
Dates, chopped, or raisins	2 tbsp.	Macadamia nuts, chopped	1 tbsp.

1. Combine boiling water, 1/2 cup milk, oats and salt in an ovenproof casserole. Let sit for 5 minutes.
2. Stir in the ginger, dates, cinnamon and 1 tbsp. of maple syrup.
3. Cover and place in 350 degrees oven for 45 minutes; remove cover for last 5 minutes of baking.
4. Drizzle 1 tbsp. of maple syrup over oatmeal, and then top with banana slices and macadamia nuts. Serve hot with 1 cup warmed milk.

Nutrition Facts

Serving Size (233g)

Amount Per Serving

Calories 310 Calories from Fat 60

	% Daily Value*
Total Fat 7g	11%
Saturated Fat 2g	10%
Trans Fat 0g	
Cholesterol 10mg	3%
Sodium 260mg	11%
Total Carbohydrate 59g	20%
Dietary Fiber 5g	20%
Sugars 28g	
Protein 9g	

Pineapple Oat Breakfast Squares

By: Alyssa Moreau

9 servings

Pineapple, fresh, cut into thin 1/2-inch pieces	2 cups
Arrowroot or cornstarch with 1 tbsp. water, optional	2 tsp.
Oats	1 1/2 cups
Whole-wheat pastry flour	1 cup
Baking powder	3/4 tsp.
Salt	1/4 tsp.
Cinnamon	1/2 tsp.
Nutmeg	1/4 tsp.
Macadamia nut oil	3 tbsp.
Pineapple juice concentrate	1/4 cup, plus 2 tbsp.
Hawaiian honey	1/4 cup
Macadamia nuts, chopped fine	2 tbsp.

1. In a saucepan, cook the pineapple on medium heat with 2 tbsp. of juice concentrate for about 10 minutes or until soft. (If there is a lot of liquid, make a slurry of arrowroot/water and add in, stirring until it thickens.)
2. Blend 1/2 cup of oats in blender or food processor to create a flour-like consistency. In a large bowl, add the processed oats with the rest of the oats and other dry ingredients (except macadamia nuts), and mix well.
3. Separately, combine the oil, juice concentrate and honey. Stir well, then add to the dry mixture. Take 2 cups of this mixture and press into a non-stick or lightly oiled 8"x8" pan.
4. Top with the pineapple, covering the whole surface with the fruit.
5. Add the macadamia nuts to the reserved oat mixture and combine. Sprinkle this evenly over the fruit and press in lightly.
6. Bake at 350 degrees for 23 to 30 minutes or when brown and crisp. Cool on rack before cutting into squares.

Tip: These squares are healthy enough to serve for breakfast, or as a nice energy booster snack.

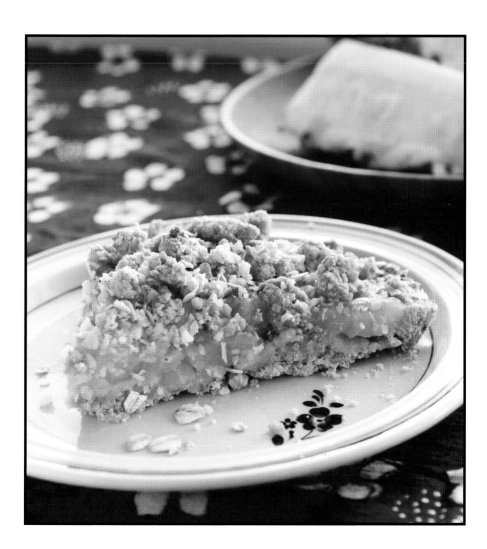

Nutrition Facts	
Serving Size (81g)	
Amount Per Serving	
Calories 210	Calories from Fat 60
	% Daily Value*
Total Fat 7g	**11%**
Saturated Fat 0.5g	**3%**
Trans Fat 0g	
Cholesterol 0mg	**0%**
Sodium 115mg	**5%**
Total Carbohydrate 34g	**11%**
Dietary Fiber 3g	**12%**
Sugars 14g	
Protein 4g	

Stuffed Hyotan (Long Squash)

By: Sharon Kobayashi

4 servings

Hyotan squash	2 lbs.	Ricotta cheese	1/4 cup
Ground turkey or		Garlic, minced	3 cloves
chicken breast (4 oz.)	1/2 cup, packed	Tomatoes, diced, including juices	1 can
Onion, minced (about 1 oz.)	2 tbsp.	Red pepper flakes	1/4 tsp.
Pine nuts, toasted	2 tbsp.	Extra-virgin olive oil	2 tbsp.
Salt	1/4 tsp.	Parmesan cheese	4 tbsp.
Italian bread crumbs	1/4 cup	Pepper	to taste
Egg whites, lightly beaten	2 each		

Fresh chopped herbs for garnish (parsley, oregano, thyme, basil)

1. Pre-heat oven to 350 degrees and boil a large pot of water.
2. Peel squash using a vegetable peeler, discard stem and end pieces.
3. Cut squash into 4 even cylindrical pieces, use a spoon to remove cores and seeds.
4. Boil squash pieces for 3 to 4 minutes to par-cook, and drain well.
5. Combine next 7 ingredients (turkey through ricotta cheese), mix well to combine.
6. Fill centers of squash pieces with turkey mixture.
7. In an oven-proof pan, add garlic, tomatoes, red pepper and olive oil.
8. Place squash in pan, top each piece with 1 tbsp. Parmesan cheese.
9. Bake approximately 45 to 60 minutes, or until squash is tender but still firm.*
10. Sprinkle with fresh herbs before serving with rice or pasta.

* Broil top if cheese does not brown, or if browning too much, cover lightly with aluminum foil.

Hyotan (long squash), is one of the many Asian squashes locally grown and available at farmers markets and Chinatown markets in Hawaiʻi. These squashes usually have firm, juicy flesh and neutral flavor, and are most amendable to stuffing and baking or steaming. The water content of the squash keeps the stuffing moist. The squash absorbs the flavor of the flavoring agents and sauce very well. So this recipe is an example for you to create a variety of dishes using Asian squashes, by varying the seasoning, flavoring agents and sauces.

Nutrition Facts	
Serving Size (355g)	
Amount Per Serving	
Calories 310	Calories from Fat 150
	% Daily Value*
Total Fat 17g	**26%**
Saturated Fat 3.5g	**18%**
Trans Fat 0g	
Cholesterol 30mg	**10%**
Sodium 480mg	**20%**
Total Carbohydrate 27g	**9%**
Dietary Fiber 5g	**20%**
Sugars 8g	
Protein 15g	

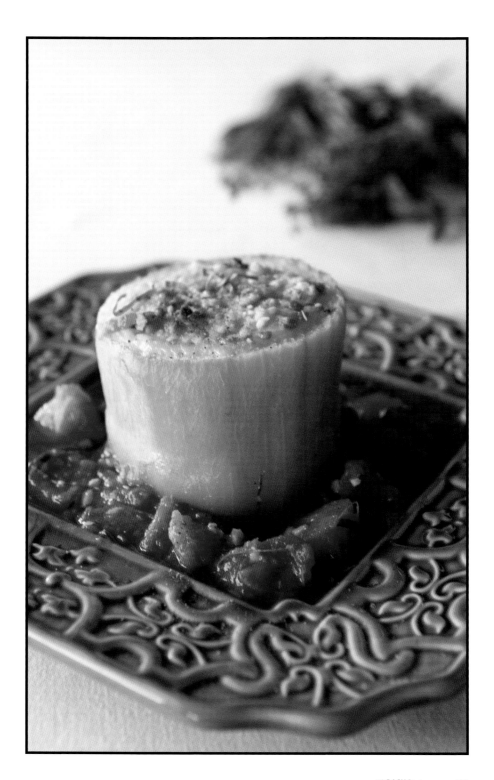

Asian-Style Curry Noodle Stir Fry

By: Alyssa Moreau

4 servings

Fresh Chinese cooked noodles, preferably Chun Wah Kam brand	1-10 oz. package	Broccoli flowerets	1 cup
Sesame oil	2 tsp.	Shiitake mushrooms, sliced	1/2 cup
Canola oil, or other light oil	1 tbsp.	Ginger, minced	1 tbsp.
Onion, sliced in half-moon shape	1/2 cup	Garlic, minced	2 tsp.
Carrot, sliced	1/2 cup	Snap peas	1/2 cup
Red bell pepper, sliced	1/2 cup	Tofu, marinated baked, sliced, (Oriental-style, White Wave brand)	1 cup

Sauce:

Vegetable broth, low-sodium, or pineapple juice	1/4 cup
Soy sauce, low-sodium, or Bragg's Liquid Aminos	1 tbsp.
Plum sauce	3 tbsp.
Curry powder	1 tsp.
Cornstarch or arrowroot	1 tbsp.

1. Combine all sauce ingredients and set aside.
2. Bring a pot of water to a boil and remove from the heat. Make sure there is enough water so noodles can be submerged completely.
3. Add the noodles; soak for about 1 minute and then drain. Toss with a bit of sesame oil and place on a serving platter.
4. Heat oil in a med-large sauté pan and add the onion. Sauté for 2 minutes, then add the carrot, red bell pepper, broccoli, shiitake mushrooms, ginger and garlic. Sauté for a few minutes, add 1/4 cup water, reduce heat and cover. Cook for about 5 minutes.
5. Remove cover and add the snap peas and tofu, along with the sauce. Stir until sauce thickens and snap peas are crisp tender.
6. Pour over noodles and serve.

Nutrition note: Most of the cooked noodle packages have a high level of sodium. But that should not keep you from using this recipe. It just means that you have to be watchful of the sodium level in the other meals you eat within the day. You can purchase marinated, baked tofu in most health stores and grocery stores.

Nutrition Facts

Serving Size (257g)

Amount Per Serving

Calories 260	Calories from Fat 90

	% Daily Value*
Total Fat 10g	15%
Saturated Fat 1g	5%
Trans Fat 0g	
Cholesterol 0mg	0%
Sodium 530mg	22%
Total Carbohydrate 28g	9%
Dietary Fiber 6g	24%
Sugars 7g	
Protein 14g	

Black Bean and Artichoke Patties with Avocado Salsa

By: Alyssa Moreau

4 servings

Olive oil	1 to 2 tbsp.	Black beans, low- or no-salt,	
Sweet Maui onion, chopped fine	1/4 cup	rinsed and drained	1-15 oz. can
Green pepper, minced	2 tbsp.	Artichoke hearts, water-packed, rinsed	
Garlic, minced	1 tsp.	and drained, chopped fine	1/2 cup
Cumin	1 tsp.	Salt	1/2 tsp.
Chili powder	1 tsp.	Cayenne	1/8 tsp.
Oregano	1/2 tsp.	Panko bread crumbs	1/4 cup
Cilantro, minced	2 tbsp.		

1. Heat oil in a medium (preferably non-stick) skillet and sauté onion and bell pepper until the onion starts to soften.
2. Add the garlic, spices and cilantro and cook for 1 minute.
3. In a separate bowl, mash the black beans with a potato masher or fork.
4. Add the artichoke hearts, cooked onion mixture, salt, cayenne and panko bread crumbs as needed to bind all ingredients together.
5. Form into 4 patties. Either pan-fry by using 1 tbsp. olive oil or bake at 350 degrees for 10 minutes each side.

Avocado Salsa:

Avocado, ripe, cubed	1 cup
Tomato, ripe, seeded and chopped fine	1 each
Black olives, chopped coarsely	2 tbsp.
Red onion, minced	1 tbsp.
Green onion, sliced thin	1 tbsp.
Garlic, minced	1/2 tsp.
Fresh lime juice	1 tbsp.
Salt	1/8 tsp.
Hot chili sauce (like Tabasco)	2 dashes

1. Combine all together and serve with patties on whole-wheat bun or pita bread.

Nutrition Facts

Serving Size (258g)

Amount Per Serving

Calories 290　　Calories from Fat 120

	% Daily Value*
Total Fat 14g	**22%**
Saturated Fat 2g	**10%**
Trans Fat 0g	
Cholesterol 0mg	**0%**
Sodium 450mg	**19%**
Total Carbohydrate 35g	**12%**
Dietary Fiber 9g	**36%**
Sugars 3g	
Protein 9g	

Spanish Rice with Napa Cabbage Rolls

By: Alyssa Moreau

4 servings

Olive oil	1 tbsp.
Sweet Maui onion, chopped	1/2 cup
Green bell pepper, chopped	1/2 cup
Garlic, minced	1 tsp.
Soy beef crumbles (Yves brand or Boca)	1 cup
Thyme	1/2 tsp.
Oregano	1/2 tsp.
Basil	1/2 tsp.
Cayenne (optional)	1/8 tsp.
Tomatoes, low-sodium, diced	1-15 oz. can
Tomato sauce, low-sodium, divided in half	1-15 oz. can
Rice, long grain, rinsed and drained	1 cup
Water	2 cups
Vinegar	2 tsp.
Parsley, chopped	2 tbsp.
Olives, ripe (optional)	1/4 cup
Salt	1/4 tsp.
Black pepper	1/4 tsp.
Napa cabbage, or won bok, steamed until soft	8 leaves
Cheddar cheese, low-fat, grated	1/2 cup

1. Heat oil in a large skillet or saucepan and sauté the onion and bell pepper for 3 to 5 minutes or until the onions start to soften.
2. Add the garlic, soy beef crumbles, herbs and cayenne. Sauté about 3 minutes.
3. Add in the diced tomatoes, 1/2 the tomato sauce, rice and water. Bring to a boil.
4. Reduce heat and cover; and cook for 20 minutes on medium-low.
5. Add the vinegar, parsley, ripe olives, salt and pepper.
6. Put this filling inside the cabbage leaves and place in a baking pan.
7. Cover the rolls with the remaining tomato sauce and grated cheese.
8. Bake 15 to 20 minutes at 350 degrees until heated through and cheese is melted.

This is a twist on the traditional "stuffed cabbage rolls" using a spicy vegetarian rendition of a local favorite—Spanish rice. Wrapped in Napa cabbage and topped with a bit of tomato sauce, melted cheese and baked, this is a dish the whole family can enjoy.

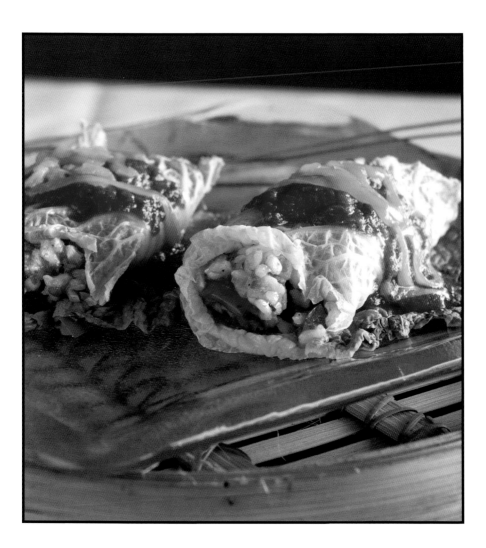

Nutrition Facts	
Serving Size (428g)	

Amount Per Serving	
Calories 360	Calories from Fat 60

	% Daily Value*
Total Fat 6g	**9**%
Saturated Fat 1.5g	**8**%
Trans Fat 0g	
Cholesterol 5mg	**2**%
Sodium 430mg	**18**%
Total Carbohydrate 57g	**19**%
Dietary Fiber 7g	**28**%
Sugars 5g	
Protein 18g	

Broccoli and Hāmākua Mushrooms with Lemongrass and Coconut Milk

By: Sharon Kobayashi

4 servings

Vegetable oil	2 tsp.
Ali'i mushrooms, sliced	4 oz .
Shallot, minced	2 each
Garlic, minced	8 cloves
Ginger, grated	2 tsp.
Jalapeño peppers, minced	2 each
Sake	1/4 cup
Japanese stock (see page 136)	1 cup
Kaffir lime leaves	2 each

Lemongrass stem, bulb split lengthwise	1 stalk
Soy sauce	4 tsp.
Carrots, sliced	2 each
Broccoli florets	1 lb.
Milk, low-fat	1 cup
Cornstarch	2 tsp.
Coconut milk	1/4 cup

Fresh chopped Thai basil, cilantro and lime juice to garnish.

1. Brown mushrooms in oil.
2. Add shallot, garlic, ginger and peppers.
3. Add sake, cook for 1 minute.
4. Add stock, lemongrass and kaffir lime leaves.
5. Bring to a boil. Reduce to simmer and cook, covered for 10 minutes.
6. Add soy sauce, carrots and broccoli. Cover and steam for 5 minutes.
7. Combine some of the milk with the cornstarch to make a slurry. Add the rest of the milk to the pot.
8. Add cornstarch/milk slurry. Bring to a boil and remove from heat.
9. Stir in coconut milk and herbs. Squeeze lime juice to taste.
10. Serve over brown rice.

Nutrition note: When making stocks with Asian ingredients, some may contain ingredients with high levels of sodium, such as dried *bonito* (fish flakes), whereas *konbu* (dried seaweed) contains natural flavor enhancers. However not all the stock will be served, so the sodium intake is actually lower than what is calculated from the ingredient list.

Nutrition Facts

Serving Size (359g)

Amount Per Serving

Calories 270	Calories from Fat 70

	% Daily Value*
Total Fat 8g	12%
Saturated Fat 4g	20%
Trans Fat 0g	
Cholesterol 20mg	7%
Sodium 460mg	19%
Total Carbohydrate 34g	11%
Dietary Fiber 8g	32%
Sugars 6g	
Protein 15g	

Crispy Spinach and Egg Cups

By: Sharon Kobayashi

6 servings

Spinach, washed, (remove root ends, blanch, squeeze dry and chop)	1 lb.	Tomato paste	1 tbsp.
Shallot, minced	2 tbsp. (1 oz.)	Dried oregano	1/2 tsp.
Garlic	2 cloves	Ricotta cheese	1/2 cup
Mushrooms, sliced thin	4 each	Eggs	6 each
Flour	1 tbsp.	Egg whites	2 each
Cajun seasoning	1/2 tsp.	Phyllo dough	6 sheets
		Salsa	6 tbsp.

1. Pre-heat oven to 350 degrees.
2. Combine first 9 ingredients (spinach through ricotta).
3. Add egg white from 2 eggs, mix thoroughly.
4. Spray a large-size muffin tin with cooking spray.
5. Spray one side of a sheet of phyllo with cooking spray.
6. Fold in half (spray side out), and half again so sheet is 1/4 size.
7. Fit into muffin tin (some of sheet will stick out). Repeat with remaining sheets.
8. Fill each cup with 1/3 cup of spinach mixture.
9. Bake for 25 minutes. Remove cups from muffin tin by gently inverting.
10. Transfer cups to a baking sheet. Crack an egg onto the top each cup.
11. Bake for 15 minutes or until egg is cooked and crust is deep brown.
12. Top each cup with 1 tbsp. of salsa and serve immediately.

Tip: After first bake (25 minutes), cups can be refrigerated or frozen for later use. Defrost overnight in refrigerator. If you prefer scrambled egg, scramble eggs in a skillet and add to cup after baking as directed.

Nutrition note: This is an example of how to balance your meals over a week's time. The cholesterol level for this recipe is at 190mg per serving, slightly higher than the DASH recommended 150mg daily nutrient goal. However, the consumption of up to 4 eggs per week keeps you within the recommended limit for the week provided that you reduce your cholesterol intake for the rest of the week.

Nutrition Facts

Serving Size (200g)

Amount Per Serving

Calories 180	Calories from Fat 60

% Daily Value*

Total Fat 7g	11%
Saturated Fat 2g	10%
Trans Fat 0g	
Cholesterol 190mg	63%
Sodium 370mg	15%
Total Carbohydrate 18g	6%
Dietary Fiber 2g	8%
Sugars 3g	
Protein 12g	

Fresh Fish Tacos with Hearts of Palm Salsa   By: Sharon Kobayashi

4 servings

Mahi mahi, (or other firm-fleshed fish), fresh, cut bite size	8 oz.
Salsa	2 tbsp.
Garlic, minced	2 cloves
Chili powder	1 tsp.
Cumin	1 tsp.
Vegetable oil	1 tsp.
Lime, juice and zest	1 each
Cilantro leaves, minced	2 tbsp.
Hearts of palm, shredded	8 oz.
Garlic, minced	1 clove
Onion, minced	2 tbsp.
Jalapeño, minced	1 to 2 each
Salt	1/2 tsp.
Avocado, Haas (or other small avocado), diced	1 each
Corn tortillas, unsalted	8 each

1. Marinate fish in salsa, garlic, spices and oil for approximately 10 minutes.
2. Combine next 7 ingredients (lime through salt) together in a bowl, reserving half the lime juice. Toss well to combine.
3. Gently toss avocado into salsa, taste and add more lime juice if needed.
4. In a hot skillet, brown fish on all sides, about 5 minutes.
5. Heat corn tortillas by steaming or in microwave, covered with a damp paper towel.

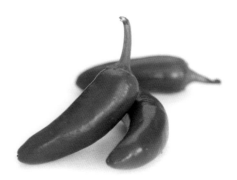

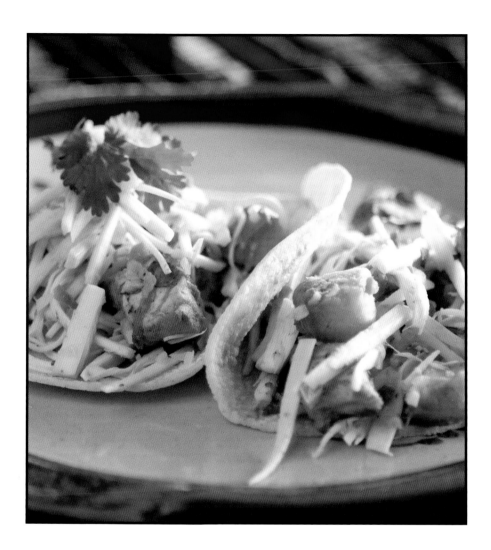

Nutrition Facts

Serving Size (255g)

Amount Per Serving

Calories 340   Calories from Fat 100

% Daily Value*

Total Fat 11g	**17**%
Saturated Fat 1.5g	**8**%
Trans Fat 0g	
Cholesterol 40mg	**13**%
Sodium 420mg	**18**%
Total Carbohydrate 48g	**16**%
Dietary Fiber 8g	**32**%
Sugars 11g	
Protein 17g	

Fritatta with Choy Sum and Goat Cheese   By: Sharon Kobayashi

6 servings

Vegetable oil	2 tsp.
Mushrooms, sliced	4 each (about 3 oz.)
Garlic	6 to 8 cloves
Choy sum, blanched, squeezed dry and chopped	1 lb.
Salt	1/2 tsp.
Egg substitute (e.g. Egg Beaters)	3/4 cup
Eggs, medium	3 each
Goat cheese (chèvre)	6 tbsp. (3 oz.)
Tomatoes, diced	2 each (about 12 oz.)
Shallot, minced	1 tsp.

1. Pre-heat oven to 400 degrees.
2. In a non-stick oven-safe pan, heat oil.
3. Sauté mushrooms until brown.
4. Add garlic, sauté briefly, add choy sum, salt, egg substitute and eggs.
5. Sprinkle top with cheese and transfer pan to oven.
6. Bake for approximately 15 minutes or until egg is set.
7. Meanwhile, mix tomatoes and shallot.
8. Top slices of fritatta with tomato mixture before serving.

Substitutions: This recipe uses a mixture of medium eggs and egg substitute. For any recipe, 1/4 cup of egg substitute is equivalent to one egg. You can also use a total of 1 1/2 cups of egg substitute instead of eggs altogether. You can substitute choy sum with other kinds of green leafy vegetables, such as spinach to create variation of flavor. Adjust the amount of minced shallot and garlic to balance the bitterness of the vegetables.

Nutrition Facts

Serving Size (210g)

Amount Per Serving

Calories 150   Calories from Fat 70

	% Daily Value*
Total Fat 8g	**12%**
Saturated Fat 4g	**20%**
Trans Fat 0g	
Cholesterol 105mg	**35%**
Sodium 380mg	**16%**
Total Carbohydrate 8g	**3%**
Dietary Fiber 1g	**4%**
Sugars 3g	
Protein 12g	

Hawai'i-Style Baked Beans

By: Alyssa Moreau

4 servings

Oil, high-oleic safflower	1 tbsp.
Sweet Maui onion, sliced thin (half-moon style)	1 cup
Mustard, dry	1 tsp.
Bay leaf	1 leaf
Cloves, whole	3 cloves
Ginger, dry	1/2 tsp.
Allspice	1/8 tsp.
Carrot, diced	1/2 cup
Garlic, minced	1 tsp.
Ginger, fresh, grated or minced	1 tsp.
Tomato, fresh, seeded and chopped	1/2 cup
Pineapple chunks with juice	1-8 oz. can
Pineapple, crushed	1-4 oz. can
Navy beans, cooked	5 cups
Rice vinegar	1 tbsp.
Soy sauce, low-sodium, or Bragg's Liquid Aminos	1 tbsp.
Molasses	2 tbsp.
Hawaiian lehua honey	1 tbsp.

1. Sauté onions and carrots in oil for a few minutes, then add the garlic, ginger and tomato.
2. Cook a few minutes more then add the dry spices.
3. Heat through a minute and add the rest of the ingredients.
4. Bring to a boil, then reduce heat and simmer, covered, for 30 minutes.

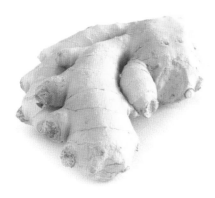

Nutrition Facts

Serving Size (534g)

Amount Per Serving

Calories 620   Calories from Fat 100

	% Daily Value*
Total Fat 11g	**17**%
Saturated Fat 2g	**10**%
Trans Fat 0g	
Cholesterol 0mg	**0**%
Sodium 230mg	**10**%
Total Carbohydrate 119g	**40**%
Dietary Fiber 37g	**148**%
Sugars 35g	
Protein 22g	

6 to 8 servings

Crust:

White flour	3/4 cup
Whole-wheat pastry flour	3/4 cup
Salt	1/4 tsp.
Baking powder	1/2 tsp.
Dill	1 tsp.
Light oil (safflower)	3 tbsp.
Water, cool	3 to 4 tbsp.

1. Combine dry ingredients in a medium bowl.
2. Mix together the wet ingredients and pour into the center of the dry ingredients.
3. Fold in until just combined.
4. Pat into a flat disk and roll into a thin round shape; place in pie plate and crimp edges.

Filling:

Tofu, (preferably Mrs. Cheng's Nigari), drained, squeezed dry with paper towels	1-20 oz. block
Olive oil	2 tbsp.
Balsamic vinegar	1 tbsp.
Rice vinegar or lemon juice, fresh	1 tbsp.
Miso, mellow white	2 tsp.
Salt	1/2 tsp.
Pepper	1/4 tsp.
Onion, finely chopped	1 medium
Red bell pepper, chopped	1/2 cup
Shiitake mushrooms, fresh, sliced	1 cup
Garlic, minced	2 cloves
Asparagus, fresh, trimmed to 4-inch pieces, (cut remaining stalks into 1/2-inch pieces for sautéing)	1/2 lb.
Parsley, fresh, chopped	1 tbsp.
Italian seasoning	1 tsp.

1. In a food processor, combine the tofu, 1 tbsp. oil, rice vinegar (or lemon juice), miso, salt, pepper. Process until smooth and creamy. Transfer to a medium bowl.
2. Sauté the vegetables and garlic (except the asparagus spears, parsley and reserve 8 slices of shiitake mushroom for decoration) in a non-stick sauté pan with remaining 1 tbsp. olive oil.
3. When the vegetables begin to soften, add in the fresh parsley and Italian seasoning. Cook 1 minute more to release flavors.
4. Add the cooked vegetables to the tofu mixture and mix well.
5. Smooth into the pie crust and decorate the top with asparagus spears (in a wheel design with shiitake mushroom slices in between). Brush a little olive oil over the spears to keep them from drying out during the baking process.
6. Bake at 350 degrees for about 35 minutes, or until the filling is firm to touch, and crust is lightly browned.
7. Serve warm or at room temperature.

This is a great way to be creative with tofu! Instead of eggs, tofu is great as a filling for quiche. This one is an eye-catcher, great for a party or special someone.

Tip: Mrs. Cheng's firm nigari tofu or Hinoichi Extra-Firm tofu have a good texture that is not too soft and wet.

Nutrition Facts	
Serving Size (221g)	
Amount Per Serving	
Calories 310	Calories from Fat 140
	% Daily Value*
Total Fat 16g	25%
Saturated Fat 2g	10%
Trans Fat 0g	
Cholesterol 0mg	0%
Sodium 400mg	17%
Total Carbohydrate 32g	11%
Dietary Fiber 5g	20%
Sugars 4g	
Protein 13g	

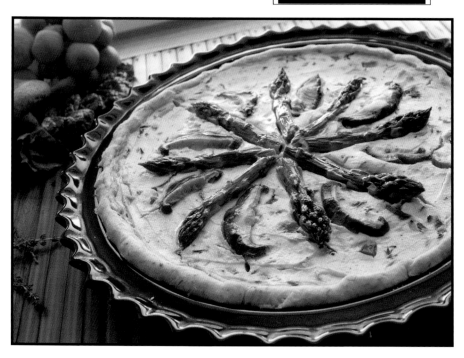

6 servings

Boca (vegetarian) burgers, chopped	2 burgers (8 to 10 oz.)	Egg replacer, dry (or 1 egg)	2 tbsp.
Canola oil	2 tbsp.	Veganaise mayo	1/3 cup
Garlic, minced	2 cloves	Salt and pepper	to taste
Ginger, minced	1 tbsp., plus 2 tsp.	Green onions, sliced thin	1 to 2 tbsp.
Stir-fry sauce (store bought)	1 tbsp., plus 1/4 cup	Bragg's Liquid Aminos, or	
Shiitake mushrooms, fresh, chopped	4 each	soy sauce, low-sodium	1 tbsp.
Carrot, grated	1 each	Sugar	1 pinch
Green beans, small pieces	1/2 cup	Arrowroot mixed with	
Water chestnuts, chopped	1/2 can	2 tbsp. water	2 tsp.
Fresh tofu, (preferably Mrs. Cheng's),		Sesame seeds, toasted,	
drained, patted dry, crumbled	1-20 oz. block	as garnish	1 tbsp.

1. Sauté the ground beef or Boca burgers in oil with the garlic, 1 tbsp. of ginger, 1 tbsp. stir-fry sauce. Mash mixture with a fork or wooden spoon.
2. Combine rest of ingredients (except 1/4 cup reserved stir-fry sauce, 2 tsp. ginger, 1 tbsp. green onions, arrowroot and sesame seeds), in a large bowl and add the ground beef/Boca burger mixture. Mix well.
3. Place mixture into a 9"x9" pan and bake at 355 degrees for 35 to 40 minutes.
4. Cool for 10 minutes.
5. In a small sauté pan, cook the rest of the ginger (2 tsp.), the rest of the green onion, and 1/4 cup reserved stir-fry sauce (may want to add a pinch of sugar if it's too salty tasting.)
6. Add arrowroot slurry and stir until thick.
7. Spread the sauce on top of the loaf. Garnish with sesame seeds.

Note: This recipe doubles well; use a 9"x13" pan and cook 45 minutes to 1 hour. The vegetarian burger can be substituted with lean ground beef, ground turkey or chicken. Some vegetarian meats have a higher sodium content than ground beef, so be sure to check the label. The arrowroot slurry can be substituted with cornstarch slurry.

Nutrition Facts

Serving Size (191g)

Amount Per Serving

Calories 270   Calories from Fat 130

	% Daily Value*
Total Fat 15g	**23%**
Saturated Fat 2.5g	**13%**
Trans Fat 0g	
Cholesterol 5mg	**2%**
Sodium 520mg	**22%**
Total Carbohydrate 16g	**5%**
Dietary Fiber 3g	**12%**
Sugars 3g	
Protein 20g	

Sesame Noodles with Kale and Edamame

By: Alyssa Moreau

2 to 3 servings

Buckwheat soba noodles	8 oz.
Kale, or other green-leaf vegetable	1 large bunch (about 1 1/2 lbs.)
Edamame (soybeans), shelled	1 cup
Toasted sesame oil	1 1/2 tbsp.
Soy sauce, low-sodium	1 tbsp.
Sesame seeds, toasted	1 tbsp.

1. Trim off thick stem from kale and slice the leaves into bite-size pieces. Place in a bowl, rinse well and drain in colander.
2. In a pot of boiling water, add noodles, edamame and kale. Be sure to submerge kale in water to cook evenly.
3. Cook for 5 minutes or until noodles are done. Kale should be tender and edamame soft.
4. Drain in a colander and rinse with cold water to cool down the noodles.
5. Shake well to release all the excess liquid caught in the kale leaves.
6. Toss the kale with toasted sesame oil and soy sauce.
7. Garnish with toasted sesame seeds. Serve hot or room temperature.

Tip: Press a chunk of fresh ginger through a garlic press to release the juice. Add ginger juice to the noodles.

Substitutions: Other green leaf vegetables can be substituted for kale, such as Shanghai cabbage, choy sum, bok choy. However, they require shorter cooking time than the kale and noodles, so check after about 2 to 3 minutes for tenderness, then remove.

Nutrition Facts

Serving Size (368g)

Amount Per Serving

Calories 530   Calories from Fat 120

	% Daily Value*
Total Fat 14g	**22%**
Saturated Fat 1g	**5%**
Trans Fat 0g	
Cholesterol 0mg	**0%**
Sodium 310mg	**13%**
Total Carbohydrate 87g	**29%**
Dietary Fiber 12g	**48%**
Sugars 3g	
Protein 22g	

Italian-Style Lemon Chicken

By: Sharon Kobayashi

6 servings

Garlic, minced	16 cloves	Extra-virgin olive oil	1 tbsp.
Lemons, juice and zest, (local		Flour	2 tbsp.
Meyer lemon or other thin-skin		Chicken broth, reduced-sodium	1-14.5 oz. can
variety preferred)	2 each	Pasta, angel hair, dried	12 oz.
Salt	1 tsp.	Broccoli florets	6 cups
Molasses	1 tbsp.	Fresh, chopped parsley and	
Rosemary, fresh, minced, leaves only	1 sprig	lemon wheels	garnish
Chicken thighs, bone in,			
skin removed	12 each		

1. Combine garlic, lemon juice and zest, salt, molasses and rosemary.
2. Marinate chicken in refrigerator overnight.
3. Pre-heat a large, stove-safe casserole dish or skillet on medium high, add oil.
4. Brown chicken pieces in batches on all sides. Reserve marinade.
5. Put browned (half-cooked) chicken in a bowl.
6. Add flour to the pan, stirring.
7. Add reserved marinade and chicken broth to the pan.
8. Bring to a boil, scraping bottom of pan to release residue at bottom.
9. Add chicken back to pan, bring to a boil. Reduce to a simmer.
10. Cook partially covered until done for 30 to 40 minutes, turning chicken halfway.
11. If sauce is too thick, add some water. If too thin, reduce after removing cooked chicken.
12. Meanwhile, boil water and cook pasta. Add broccoli at the last minute.
13. Drain pasta and broccoli, mix with sauce and serve with chicken.
14. Garnish with chopped fresh parsley and lemon wheels, if desired.

Tip: Chicken thighs are more flavorful and have a better texture than chicken breasts. They also contain more moisture and are better for sautéing and braising without drying out as fast. On average, each thigh contains about 2 oz. of meat.

Nutrition Facts

Serving Size (414g)

Amount Per Serving

Calories 530   Calories from Fat 80

	% Daily Value*
Total Fat 9g	**14%**
Saturated Fat 1.5g	**8%**
Trans Fat 0g	
Cholesterol 95mg	**32%**
Sodium 540mg	**23%**
Total Carbohydrate 76g	**25%**
Dietary Fiber 5g	**20%**
Sugars 5g	
Protein 38g	

Kabocha Pumpkin Stew
By: Alyssa Moreau

4 servings

Light oil	2 tsp.
Kabocha pumpkin, cut into 1-inch pieces	2 cups
Garlic, minced	2 tbsp.
Ginger, minced	1 1/2 tsp.
Vegetable broth, low-sodium, or water	1 can
Soy sauce, low-salt	1 tbsp.
Mirin	2 tbsp.
Potato, cut into 1-inch pieces, partially cooked	1 cup
Carrot, large, cut into 1-inch pieces	1 cup
Shiitake mushrooms, fresh, sliced	1/2 cup
Kombu (dried seaweed) ties*	1 cup (or more to taste)
Aburage (deep-fried tofu),** optional	1 package (about 1 cup)
Water chestnuts, sliced	1 can (about 1/2 cup)

1. Sauté kabocha in heated oil until lightly browned. Add garlic and ginger, then sauté 1 minute.
2. Add rest of ingredients and simmer for about 30 minutes or until the kabocha is soft.

*pre-soaked, tied into knots 3 inches apart and cut into pieces
** par-boiled to remove the oil, then cut into pieces

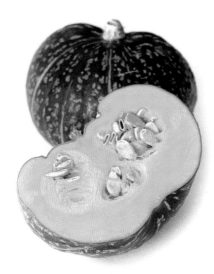

Nutrition Facts
Serving Size (314g)

Amount Per Serving

Calories 210   Calories from Fat 70

	% Daily Value*
Total Fat 8g	**12%**
Saturated Fat 1g	**5%**
Trans Fat 0g	
Cholesterol 0mg	**0%**
Sodium 170mg	**7%**
Total Carbohydrate 29g	**10%**
Dietary Fiber 5g	**20%**
Sugars 7g	
Protein 7g	

4 servings

Udon noodles, cooked (preferably dry-style Hula brand)	12 oz.
Sesame oil	2 tsp.
Won bok cabbage, sliced thin	4 cups
Carrot, grated	1/2 cup
Red bell pepper, sliced thin	1/2 cup
Japanese cucumber, seeded, sliced in 1/2-moon pieces	1 cup
Mint, chopped	1/2 cup
Cilantro, chopped	1/2 cup
Green onion, chopped	1/2 cup
Tofu, marinated, baked (Oriental style, White Wave brand), optional	1 cup

1. Cook udon noodles about 8 minutes; drain and rinse under cool water until at room temperature.
2. Toss with a bit of sesame oil to prevent sticking.
3. Combine the rest of the salad ingredients in a large bowl and add in the noodles. Toss well.

Dressing:

Garlic, minced	2 cloves	Honey	2 tbsp.
Ginger, fresh, minced	1 tbsp.	Sambal chile paste	1/4 tsp.
Peanut butter, smooth,		Soy sauce, low-sodium	1 tbsp.
non-hydrogenated	1/4 cup	Rice vinegar	1 tbsp.
Silken tofu, firm (Mori-Nu brand)	1/2 cup	Water (as needed)	1/2 to 1 cup

1. Place all ingredients (except water) in blender.
2. Add 1/2 cup water then blend, adding more as necessary to get a preferred consistency.

To serve, place salad on plates and serve dressing on the side.

Tip: This is a crunchy salad, with some chilled noodles mixed in. The peanut sauce is "lightened" calorie-wise by adding silken tofu without compromising the flavor. With some marinated tofu added in, it is substantial enough to serve as an entree at lunch; also great to take to potlucks.

Nutrition Facts	
Serving Size (342g)	
Amount Per Serving	
Calories 390	Calories from Fat 130
	% Daily Value*
Total Fat 14g	**22%**
Saturated Fat 2g	**10%**
Trans Fat 0g	
Cholesterol 0mg	**0%**
Sodium 440mg	**18%**
Total Carbohydrate 41g	**14%**
Dietary Fiber 4g	**16%**
Sugars 12g	
Protein 20g	

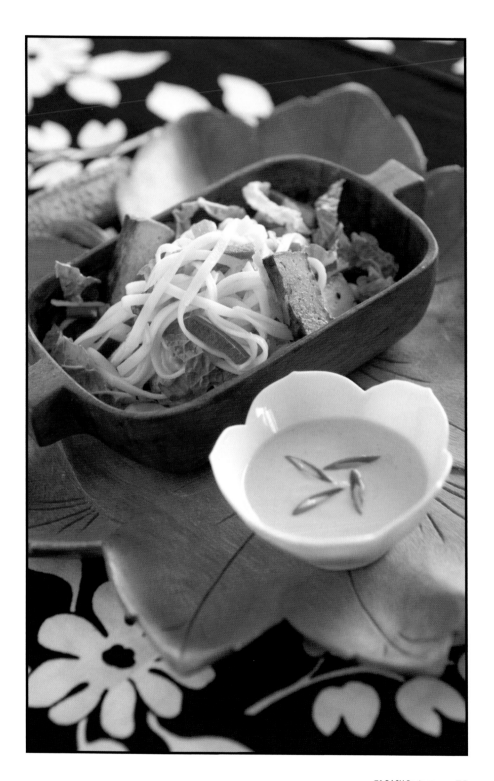

Local-Style Hamburger Patties

5 servings

Shiitake mushrooms, dried	2 each
Beef broth, reduced-sodium	1 cup
Vegetable oil	1 tsp.
Onions, 1/4" dice	1 cup
Celery, 1/4" dice	2 stalks
Mushrooms, fresh, sliced	8 oz.
Garlic, minced	3 cloves
Tomato paste	1 tbsp.
Bread, processed into crumbs	1 slice (about 3 oz.)
Hamburger, extra lean	10 oz.
Egg	1 each
Worcestershire sauce	1 tbsp.
Green onion, minced	2 stalks

1. Rehydrate dried shiitake mushrooms in warm beef broth. Mince mushrooms.
2. In a skillet, sauté onions, celery and mushrooms until tender. Add garlic and tomato paste. Sauté 1 to 2 more minutes.
3. Add beef broth and fresh mushrooms.
4. Cook until most of the broth is evaporated. Cool mixture.
5. Pre-heat oven to 400 degrees.
6. Add rest of ingredients and mix well to combine.
7. Portion mixture into 5 pieces and form into patties.
8. Spray a baking sheet with cooking spray.
9. Bake patties about 15 to 20 minutes, flip over halfway through.

Serving suggestion: Serve with mushroom gravy (see page 137) or make a sandwich with 1 tbsp. light mayonnaise and shredded cabbage. This is a low-fat burger. The mixture of minced sautéed mushrooms adds moisture to the beef patties in place of fat, and allows them to be baked without drying out.

Nutrition Facts

Serving Size (267g)

Amount Per Serving	
Calories 150	Calories from Fat 45

	% Daily Value*
Total Fat 5g	8%
Saturated Fat 1.5g	8%
Trans Fat 0g	
Cholesterol 75mg	25%
Sodium 180mg	8%
Total Carbohydrate 12g	4%
Dietary Fiber 2g	8%
Sugars 4g	
Protein 17g	

Macadamia Furikake-Crusted Tofu

By: Alyssa Moreau

4 servings

Firm tofu (preferably Mrs. Cheng's or Hinoichi brand), drained, dried and sliced into 8 pieces	1-20 oz. block
Sesame oil, light	1 to 2 tbsp.
Black sesame seeds	1 tbsp.
Sesame seeds, toasted	2 tbsp.
Macadamia nuts, finely ground	2 tbsp.
Sea salt	1/4 tsp.
Nori (dried seaweed), shredded	1/4 cup

Nutrition Facts

Serving Size (169g)

Amount Per Serving

Calories 280 Calories from Fat 170

	% Daily Value*
Total Fat 19g	29%
Saturated Fat 2.5g	13%
Trans Fat 0g	
Cholesterol 0mg	0%
Sodium 400mg	17%
Total Carbohydrate 9g	3%
Dietary Fiber 3g	12%
Sugars 0g	
Protein 22g	

1. Mix seeds, nuts, salt and nori together in a small bowl.
2. Brush tofu slices lightly with oil and dip into the seed/nut/nori mix to coat the top.
3. Lightly oil a baking sheet and place tofu slices on it.
4. Bake at 350 degrees for about 30 minutes or until browned and crisp.

Honey Teriyaki Chicken Bowl

By: Sharon Kobayashi

4 servings

Chicken thighs, boneless and skinless	1 lb.	Sesame seeds	1 tbsp.
Soy sauce	2 tsp.	Green onion, chopped	2 stalks
Hawaiian honey	2 tsp.	Sesame oil	1 tsp.
Ginger, fresh, grated	1 tsp.	Vegetable fried rice (see page 82)	4 cups
Garlic, minced	4 cloves		
Molasses	1 tsp.		
Worcestershire sauce	1 tsp.		

1. Mix 1 tsp. soy sauce with 1 tsp. honey, set aside.
2. Add the rest of the ingredients together, marinate chicken thighs for 2 hours.
3. Broil or grill chicken, slice.
4. While hot, toss with reserved soy sauce and honey mixture.
5. Serve over steamed or vegetable fried rice.

Nutrition Facts

Serving Size (108g)

Amount Per Serving

Calories 240 Calories from Fat 140

	% Daily Value*
Total Fat 16g	25%
Saturated Fat 4g	20%
Trans Fat 0g	
Cholesterol 75mg	25%
Sodium 180mg	8%
Total Carbohydrate 6g	2%
Dietary Fiber 0g	0%
Sugars 4g	
Protein 16g	

Loco Moco Fried Rice

By: Sharon Kobayashi

6 servings

Vegetable fried rice (see recipe below)	5 cups
Beef, ground, extra lean	6 oz.
Beef broth, reduced-sodium	1/2 cup
Eggs, medium, poached	6 each
Sweet Maui onion and mushroom gravy (see page 137)	3/4 cup

1. Prepare vegetable fried rice as directed.
2. In a non-stick pan, brown beef, breaking it up into small pieces.
3. Add beef broth, scraping bottom of pan until liquid is nearly evaporated.
4. Add fried rice and toss to combine.
5. Serve rice topped with 1 egg and 2 tbsp. gravy.

Tip: If cooking for a few people, portion and freeze extra fried rice after cooling. You can also use 1 oz. beef and 1 tbsp. beef broth to 3/4 cup vegetable fried rice for a single portion.

Nutrition note: This is an example for balancing your cholesterol intake while eating the food that you desire. The cholesterol level for one serving of this meal is above the DASH daily nutrition goal. This means you should ensure that the other meals within the same and next day are low in cholesterol. You can still enjoy a local favorite while staying within the eating plan's weekly goal. Another alternative is using just the egg white.

Vegetable Fried Rice

5 servings

Shiitake mushroom, dried	2 each	Cabbage, shredded	4 oz.
Seaweed, hijiki, dried	1 tbsp.	Soy sauce	3 tsp.
Water, hot	1/2 cup	Worcestershire sauce	1 tsp.
Vegetable oil	2 tsp.	Brown rice, day-old	3 cups
Burdock and carrots, frozen, julienne	4 oz. each	Green onion	2 stalks
Daikon, julienne	4 oz.		

1. Soak mushroom and seaweed in hot water for about 10 minutes.
2. Remove mushroom from water. Squeeze mushrooms over soaking container and chop.

Recipe continues on next page.

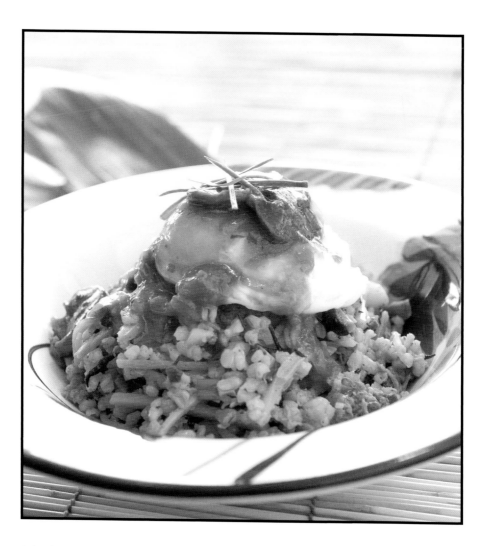

3. In a hot pan, sauté vegetables (except green onions) until wilted.
4. Add soy sauce and Worcestershire sauce to hijiki and soaking liquids.
5. Add rice to pan and sauté briefly. Add hijiki, liquids and green onion to the pan.
6. Cook, stirring, until liquid is evaporated.

Nutrition Facts

Serving Size (318g)

Amount Per Serving	
Calories 280	Calories from Fat 90

	% Daily Value*
Total Fat 10g	**15%**
Saturated Fat 2.5g	**13%**
Trans Fat 0g	
Cholesterol 205mg	**68%**
Sodium 280mg	**12%**
Total Carbohydrate 32g	**11%**
Dietary Fiber 3g	**12%**
Sugars 3g	
Protein 16g	

Salmon with Lomi Lomi Tomato

By: Sharon Kobayashi

4 servings

Salmon fillet, skin on	1 lb.
Tomato, 1/4" dice	4 each
Onion, 1/2" dice	1 each
Salt	1/2 tsp.
Lemon juice	1 to 2 tbsp.
Green onion, chopped	1 to 2 stalks

1. Combine tomatoes, onions, salt, lemon juice and green onion.
2. Mix and refrigerate at least 1 hour before using.
3. Pre-heat a non-stick skillet on medium high.
4. Add salmon (skin side down), reduce heat to medium-low.
5. Cook until 3/4 done (skin should be crisp), about 6 to 8 minutes.
6. Flip fish over and finish cooking.
7. Serve salmon (skin side up) over tomato mixture, with 1/2 cup poi on the side.

This is a variation of the lomi lomi salmon that people in Hawai'i are so familiar with. The salt draws out the juice and liquid from the tomatoes and onion, which serves as a relish for the salmon. Lime juice and seasoned salt can be substituted for the plain salt and lemon juice to create different flavors. Locally-grown, bright red vine-ripened tomatoes and green onions make this a very colorful dish.

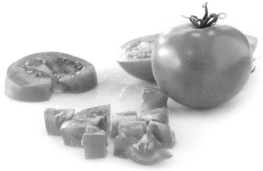

Nutrition Facts

Serving Size (248g)

Amount Per Serving

Calories 190	Calories from Fat 70

	% Daily Value*
Total Fat 7g	11%
Saturated Fat 1g	5%
Trans Fat 0g	
Cholesterol 60mg	20%
Sodium 350mg	15%
Total Carbohydrate 7g	2%
Dietary Fiber 2g	8%
Sugars 4g	
Protein 24g	

Smoky Turkey Chili with Okinawan Sweet Potato

6 servings

By: Sharon Kobayashi

Vegetable oil	1 tbsp.	Salsa	1/4 cup
Medium onion, diced small	2 each	Light beer	12 oz.
Bell pepper, diced small	2 each	Chicken broth, reduced-sodium	1 can
Celery, diced small	1 stalk	Water	1 cup
Garlic cloves, minced	4 each	Sweet potato, diced	1 lb.
Ground turkey	8 oz.	Salt	1 tsp.
Chili powder	1 to 2 tbsp.	Black beans, salt-free, drained	
Cumin	2 tsp.	and rinsed	1 can
Bay leaves	2 each	Liquid smoke	1 tsp.
Flour	2 tbsp.	Peanut butter	1 tbsp.
Tomato paste	2 tbsp.	Cheddar cheese, reduced-fat	6 tbsp.

Optional: shredded iceberg lettuce and fresh tomatoes for garnish

1. Reserve 1/4 cup onion and bell pepper. Sauté the remaining onion, pepper and celery in oil until light brown.
2. Add garlic and turkey, sauté until turkey is cooked through.
3. Add spices and flour, stir to combine.
4. Add tomato paste, peanut butter, and then stir to combine.
5. Add salsa, beer, chicken broth and water, and then bring to a boil, stirring.
6. Add sweet potato, salt, beans and liquid smoke.
7. Reduce to simmer, cook until potatoes are tender (about 20 minutes).
8. At the last 5 minutes, add reserved onion and bell pepper.
9. Top with 1 tbsp. cheddar cheese and serve with 1/2 cup brown rice.

Tip: Make chili bowls (with rice on the bottom) in freezer- and microwave-safe containers to take to work.

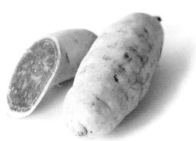

Nutrition Facts
Serving Size (430g)

Amount Per Serving

Calories 320   Calories from Fat 80

	% Daily Value*
Total Fat 9g	**14%**
Saturated Fat 2g	**10%**
Trans Fat 0g	
Cholesterol 30mg	**10%**
Sodium 670mg	**28%**
Total Carbohydrate 42g	**14%**
Dietary Fiber 9g	**36%**
Sugars 7g	
Protein 17g	

6 servings

Flank steak, lean	1 lb.
Olive oil	2 tsp.
Light beer	12 oz.
Beef broth, reduced-sodium (add water to cover, about 3 cups)	4 cups
Cloves, ground	1/4 tsp.
Cinnamon, ground	1 tsp.
Black beans, low-sodium, rinsed and drained	1 can
Onions, medium, julienne	2 each
Garlic	4 cloves
Capers, in brine , drained	1/4 cup
Tomatoes, julienne	4 each
Zucchini, julienne	3 each (about 12 oz.)
Bell peppers, sweet, large, julienne	4 each
Garlic chives (nira), cut into 2-inch lengths	4 bunches

1. Cut steak into 6 even size pieces.
2. Add 2 tsp. oil to an 8 quart pot and brown the meat on both sides.
3. Add beer, scraping bottom of pot clean, add broth, water and spices.
4. Bring to a boil, cover and reduce to simmer.
5. When meat is tender (approximately 90 minutes), remove from pot and shred meat with 2 forks.
6. Return to pot with black beans, onions, garlic and capers, cook 15 minutes.
7. Add tomatoes, zucchinis, sweet bell peppers and chives and cook until just tender, about 5 minutes.

Optional: Garnish with shredded iceberg lettuce, cilantro, minced jalapeño peppers and a squeeze of lime. Suggest serving with brown rice.

Tip: Nira is the flat Asian variety of chive. They are grown in Hawai'i and are available at most farmers' markets and Chinatown markets. Chives, like all fresh herbs, should be added last in the cooking process so their fragrance will not be cooked off. Flank steak is one of the lean cuts of meat, best for low-fat recipes.

Nutrition Facts

Serving Size (683g)

Amount Per Serving

Calories 280   Calories from Fat 70

	% Daily Value*
Total Fat 7g	11%
Saturated Fat 2g	10%
Trans Fat 0g	
Cholesterol 25mg	8%
Sodium 410mg	17%
Total Carbohydrate 27g	9%
Dietary Fiber 9g	36%
Sugars 10g	
Protein 27g	

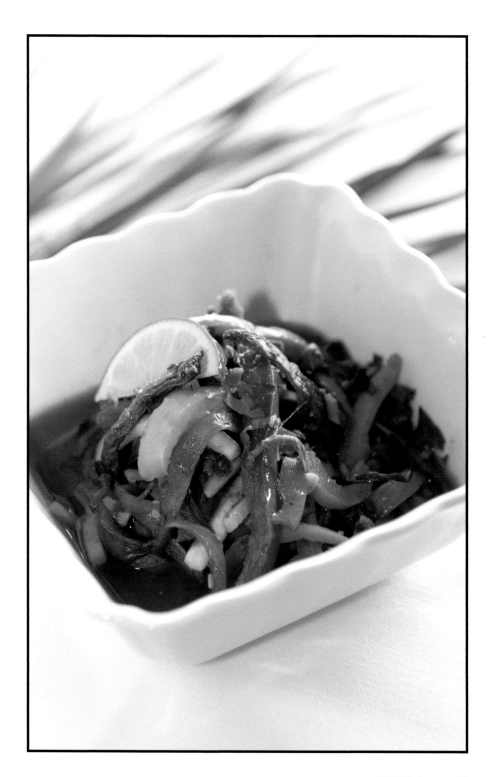

Four-Seeded Salmon with Kabocha Miso Risotto

By: Sharon Kobayashi

4 servings

Salmon fillet, cut into 4 pieces	1 lb.
Soy sauce	2 tsp.
Sesame seeds	2 tbsp.
Black mustard seeds	1/2 tsp.
Poppy seeds	1 tsp.
Fennel seeds	1/2 tsp.
Vegetable oil	2 tsp.

1. Marinate salmon in soy sauce for 10 minutes.
2. Mix seeds together, pour onto a plate.
3. Dredge one side of each salmon fillet in seed mix, thoroughly coating one side.
4. Heat oil in pan on medium, place salmon seed side down in hot pan.
5. Cook until seeds start to brown (about 3 minutes) and flip over.
6. Pour marinating juices into the pan and cook until juices evaporate.
7. Continue to cook until brown and just cooked through (4 to 8 minutes).

Tip: If need to reduce sodium further, substitute reduced-sodium soy sauce.

Nutrition note: This dish is slightly higher in cholesterol, which comes from the oil in the salmon. Remember that all foods have varying amounts of nutrients. Some we try to limit such as sodium, cholesterol and saturated fats, while others we try to increase in our diet, such as fiber, monounsaturated (olive and canola) oils and polyunsaturated (flax products, fish) oils that contain other beneficial nutrients such as the omega-3 fats in the salmon fish oil.

Kabocha Risotto with Miso

4 servings

Japanese stock (see page 136)	4 cups
Kabocha pumpkin, diced 1/2-inch cubes (about 2 cups)	8 oz.
Hot water (as needed)	1 to 2 cups
Vegetable oil	1 tsp.
Arborio rice	3/4 cup
Sake	1/4 cup
Garlic chives, diced	1/4 cup
Miso, white (dissolved in 1/4 cup cold water)	1 tbsp.

1. Cook kabocha in stock until just tender, strain reserving stock and kabocha separately.
2. Heat reserved stock until hot, but not boiling.
3. In a large heavy-bottomed sauté pan, sauté rice in vegetable oil, 1 minute.
4. Add sake to pan, stirring.
5. Add stock 1/2 cup at a time, stirring after each addition until absorbed.
6. If rice is still not cooked, add hot water as needed, 1/2 cup at a time.
7. Rice is done when grains are a little firm and sauce is creamy (about 20 to 30 minutes).
8. Add garlic chives and kabocha.
9. Remove pan from heat and stir in miso and water. Serve immediately.

Nutrition Facts

Serving Size (508g)

Amount Per Serving	
Calories 360	Calories from Fat 120

	% Daily Value*
Total Fat 14g	**22%**
Saturated Fat 1.5g	**8%**
Trans Fat 0g	
Cholesterol 65mg	**22%**
Sodium 400mg	**17%**
Total Carbohydrate 26g	**9%**
Dietary Fiber 2g	**8%**
Sugars 2g	
Protein 29g	

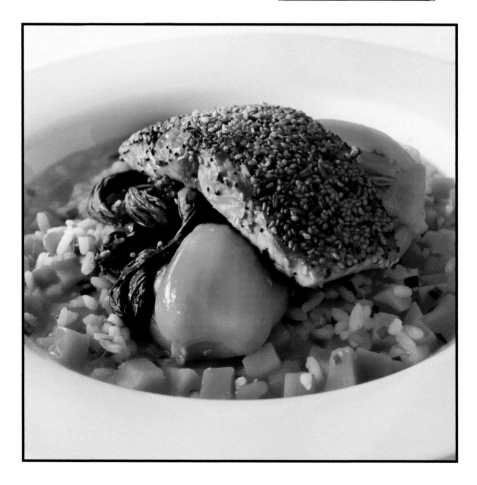

Poached Fish with Curly Cress
By: Sharon Kobayashi

4 servings

Fish fillets, cut into 4 pieces (mild fish, such as onaga, mahi mahi)	1 lb.
Lemon, sliced	1 each
Basic Asian Vinaigrette (see below)	5 tbsp.
Vegetable oil	1 tbsp.
Curly cress,* loosely measured	4 cups

1. Bring water and lemon slices (poaching liquid**) to a boil in a deep pan.
2. Add fish, cover and turn off heat.
3. Let sit, covered, until cooked through, about 10 minutes, drain and pat dry.
4. Combine vinaigrette and oil.
5. Mix vinaigrette with greens, pile on fish.
6. Serve immediately with brown rice.

Basic Asian Vinaigrette:

Shallots, fresh, chopped	1 tbsp.
Balsamic vinegar	1/4 cup
Ginger, fresh, minced	1/2 tsp.
Toasted sesame oil	1 tsp.
Soy sauce, low-sodium	1 tbsp.
Black pepper, ground	to taste

1. Combine all ingredients. Stir well before using.

*Curly cress can be substituted with other **baby greens** (young salad greens), such as baby shinkiku or baby mizuna that impart a slightly bitter note to counter the acidity of the vinaigrette. The young salad greens produced by Hawai'i farmers have bright and intense flavors due to the Islands' climate and rich soil, and can easily liven up a simple dish.

The **poaching liquid can be water or low-sodium, low-fat chicken broth flavored with a varying combination of aromatic herbs, such as cilantro or lemongrass. It takes practice to poach fish without overcooking. Poaching time depends on the thickness of the fish. The best way to test for doneness is by pressing down on the fish to check its firmness.

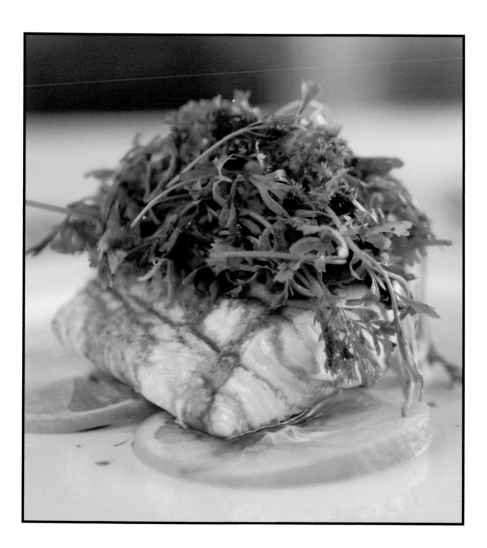

Nutrition Facts

Serving Size (156g)

Amount Per Serving

Calories 170   Calories from Fat 50

% Daily Value*

Total Fat 6g	**9%**
Saturated Fat 1g	**5%**
Trans Fat 0g	
Cholesterol 40mg	**13%**
Sodium 210mg	**9%**
Total Carbohydrate 4g	**1%**
Dietary Fiber 0g	**0%**
Sugars 2g	
Protein 24g	

Sweet Sour Won Bok Rolls

By: Alyssa Moreau

4 to 5 servings

Tofu (preferably Mrs. Cheng's), drained, hand-crumbled	1-20 oz. block	Fresh garlic, minced	1 tsp.
Green onions, chopped	2 tbsp.	Salt	1/2 tsp.
Chinese parsley, chopped	2 tbsp.	Pepper	1/8 tsp.
Shiitake mushrooms, fresh, chopped	2 tbsp.	Veganaise mayonnaise (has no egg in it)	1 tbsp.
Water chestnuts, chopped	1/4 cup	Won bok* leaves, large, blanched, cooled	10 pieces
Carrot, grated	1/4 cup	Macadamia nut oil	1 tbsp.
Fresh ginger, minced	1 tbsp.		

Glaze:

Pineapple juice, canned	1/2 cup	Soy sauce, low-sodium	1 tbsp.
Mirin	1 tbsp.	Chinese parsley, chopped	1 tbsp.
Arrowroot or cornstarch diluted in 1 tbsp. cool water to make slurry	2 tsp.	Sesame seeds, toasted	2 tsp.

1. Combine the tofu, green onions, Chinese parsley, shiitake mushrooms, water chestnuts, carrot, ginger, garlic, salt, pepper and mayonnaise. Mix well.
2. Divide into 10 portions and place each portion inside of a won bok leaf. Roll up burrito-style.
3. Heat oil in a non-stick skillet, at medium heat, sauté the won bok bundles on each side until lightly yellowed.
4. Add 1/4 cup water, bring to a boil and cover skillet. Lower heat and let steam for about 5 minutes or until heated through.
5. Take off lid and cook until water evaporates. Place on serving platter.
6. In a saucepan, combine the pineapple juice, mirin, soy sauce and arrowroot slurry, and then mix well. Bring to a boil; reduce heat and stir until thickened.
7. Pour sauce over rolls on platter.
8. Garnish top of rolls with Chinese parsley and toasted sesame seeds.

*Won bok can be substituted with Napa cabbage.

Nutrition Facts

Serving Size (300g)

Amount Per Serving

Calories 220	Calories from Fat 90

% Daily Value*

Total Fat 10g	**15%**
Saturated Fat 1.5g	**8%**
Trans Fat 0g	
Cholesterol 0mg	**0%**
Sodium 490mg	**20%**
Total Carbohydrate 14g	**5%**
Dietary Fiber 4g	**16%**
Sugars 7g	
Protein 18g	

Tofu Brunch Scrambler

By: Alyssa Moreau

3 to 4 servings

Macadamia nut oil	1 tbsp.
Sweet Maui onion, sliced thin	1/2 cup
Carrot, julienne	1/4 cup
Red bell pepper, chopped	1/4 cup
Tomato, seeded and chopped	1/2 cup
Cumin	1/2 tsp.
Oregano	1/2 tsp.
Tofu, fresh, rinsed, drained, patted dry	16 oz.
Turmeric	1/2 tsp.
Salt	1/4 tsp.
Black pepper	1/4 tsp.
Bragg's Liquid Aminos, or soy sauce, low-sodium	1 tbsp.
Peas, frozen, or fresh snap peas	1/2 cup
Tabasco	1/4 tsp.
Cheese, 2% jack or cheddar, grated	1/4 cup
Cilantro, fresh, minced	2 tbsp.

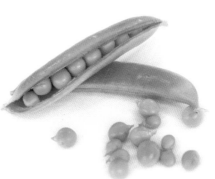

1. Heat oil in a large skillet and add the onion. Sauté for a few minutes until it starts to become soft.
2. Add the carrot and red bell pepper, and then continue to cook for about 3 minutes.
3. Add the tomatoes, cumin and oregano and heat a few minutes more.
4. Crumble the tofu into the pan, then sprinkle the turmeric, salt, pepper and Bragg's over the tofu and mix in well.
5. Add the peas and Tabasco and top with cheese.
6. Reduce heat and cover for 3 minutes or until cheese melts.
7. Serve topped with cilantro.

Tip: This is definitely a breakfast or lunch (brunch) dish. The cheese is optional. Great with a side of steamed rice.

Nutrition Facts

Serving Size (229g)

Amount Per Serving

Calories 200   Calories from Fat 110

	% Daily Value*
Total Fat 12g	18%
Saturated Fat 2g	10%
Trans Fat 0g	
Cholesterol 0mg	0%
Sodium 380mg	16%
Total Carbohydrate 10g	3%
Dietary Fiber 4g	16%
Sugars 4g	
Protein 16g	

Tofu Burgers with Mango Chutney — By: Alyssa Moreau

4 to 6 servings

Olive oil	2 tsp., plus 1 tbsp.	Light mayonnaise, or	
Onion, chopped fine	1/2 cup	Veganaise	1 tbsp.
Mushrooms or zucchini,		Panko	1 cup
chopped fine	1/2 cup	Rolled oats (more if needed)	1/2 cup
Celery, chopped fine	1/2 cup	Salt	1/2 tsp.
Carrot, grated	1/2 cup	Prepared mustard	1/2 tbsp.
Red bell pepper, chopped fine	1/2 cup	Cumin	1 tsp.
Italian parsley, fresh, minced	2 tbsp.	Curry powder	1/2 tsp.
Tofu, firm (drained and dried		Cayenne	1/2 tsp.
well), mashed	20 oz.	Mango Chutney (see page 138)	
Egg replacer (Ener-G brand),			
dry, with 2 tbsp. water, or			
equivalent to 1 egg	1 tbsp.		

1. In 2 tsp. of olive oil, sauté all the vegetables, including parsley, until soft.
2. Place in a large mixing bowl.
3. Add remaining ingredients and mix thoroughly. Add enough rolled oats to form a fairly stiff batter to form patties with your hand.
4. Form patties and sauté** in non-stick pan in 1 tbsp. olive oil.
5. Turn after a few minutes to brown both sides.

***Nutrition note:** You can use up to 2 medium eggs, which brings the cholesterol level to 75mg., while still remaining within half of your DASH daily recommended nutrient goal. If you do not want to use eggs at all, egg replacer is available in health food stores.

***Optional:** Place patties on parchment paper-lined baking sheet and bake 15 minutes each side or until lightly browned and firm to touch.

Tip: For tofu lovers, these burgers are great served in pita bread or hamburger buns with a side salad. Fresh mango chutney (see page 138) tastes delicious on top, as well as crisp cucumber, Mānoa lettuce and local tomatoes.

Substitutions: A firm tofu like Mrs. Cheng's Nigari or House of H extra firm helps to bind the burgers. If you cannot get fresh mangoes to make chutney, fresh peaches can be substituted. Veganaise mayonnaise can be found at any local health food store and can be used instead of mayonnaise.

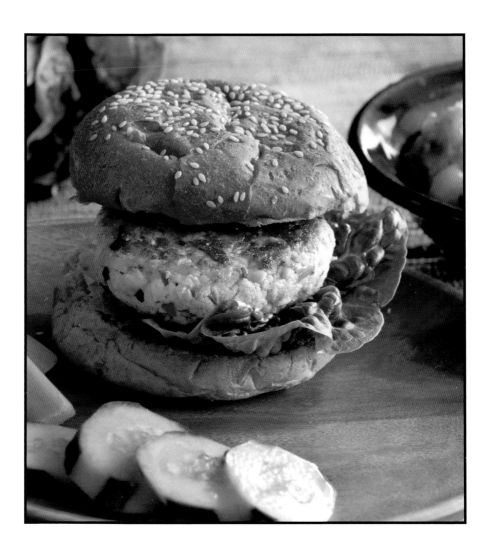

Nutrition Facts

Serving Size (207g)

Amount Per Serving

Calories 300 Calories from Fat 120

% Daily Value*

Total Fat 14g	**22%**
Saturated Fat 2g	**10%**
Trans Fat 0g	
Cholesterol 0mg	**0%**
Sodium 370mg	**15%**
Total Carbohydrate 29g	**10%**
Dietary Fiber 4g	**16%**
Sugars 3g	
Protein 17g	

Sesame (Soy) Chicken and Edamame Stir-Fry over Soba Noodles or Brown Rice

By: Alyssa Moreau

3 to 4 servings

Buckwheat soba noodles	1-8 oz. package
Light oil (canola, vegetable)	1 tbsp.
Soy chicken cutlets*	2 cups
Red bell pepper, sliced	1/2 cup
Fresh ginger, minced	1 tbsp.
Lemongrass, minced	1 stalk
Garlic, minced	2 clove
Mirin	2 tbsp.
Toasted sesame oil	1 tbsp.
Soy sauce, low-sodium, or Bragg's Liquid Aminos	2 tbsp.
Edamame (soybeans), fresh or frozen, cooked, shelled	1 cup
Snap peas	1/2 cup
Green onions, sliced	1/4 cup
Black sesame seeds, toasted (for garnish)	1 tbsp.

1. Cook noodles as directed on the package. Rinse and drain well. Toss with a little sesame oil and salt or low-sodium soy sauce. Set aside.
2. While noodles are cooking, start the stir-fry.
3. Heat oil in a sauté pan and cook the soy chicken and red bell pepper until the cutlets strips start to brown and bell peppers begin to soften.
4. Add in the ginger, lemongrass and garlic and cook for 1 minute.
5. Add mirin, toasted sesame oil, and low-sodium soy sauce and mix in well.
6. Add in the edamame, snap peas and green onions. Cook a few minutes or until the snap peas are crisp-tender. (Covering the pan works well to quicken the process.)
7. Serve over soba noodles.
8. Garnish with toasted black sesame seeds.

* Soy chicken cutlets are made from soy-based products. They are found at most health food stores, and resemble diced, cooked chicken in consistency and appearance. This is a dish where you can create variations of texture, flavor and color with different types of vegetables or starches, such as ramen, rice noodles, white or brown rice, etc.

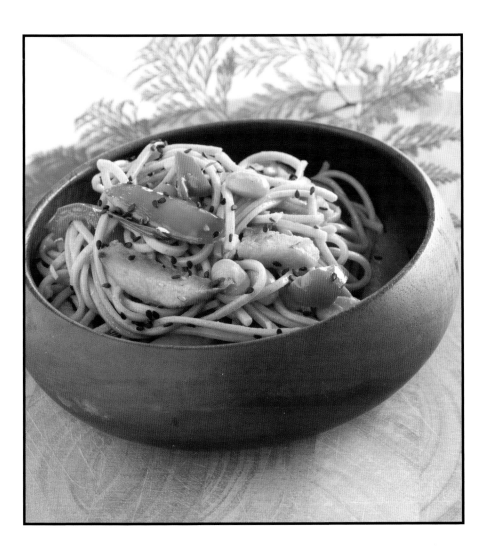

Nutrition Facts

Serving Size (263g)

Amount Per Serving

Calories 630   Calories from Fat 120

% Daily Value*

Total Fat 14g	**22%**
Saturated Fat 1g	**5%**
Trans Fat 0g	
Cholesterol 0mg	**0%**
Sodium 510mg	**21%**
Total Carbohydrate 100g	**33%**
Dietary Fiber 10g	**40%**
Sugars 8g	
Protein 28g	

Tofu Lemongrass Curry By: Alyssa Moreau

4 servings

Tofu, fresh (preferably Aloha Brand, firm)	1-16 oz.	Carrot, peeled and cut into large chunks (reserve 2 chunks for sauce)	2 cups
Canola oil	1 tbsp.	Moloka'i sweet potato, peeled and cut into large chunks	2 cups
Turmeric	sprinkle	Yukon gold potato, large, peeled and cut into chunks	1 cup
Curry powder	1/2 tsp.	Canola oil	1 tbsp.
Hawaiian salt	1/4 tsp.		
Sweet Maui onion, large chunks	1 cup		

Sauce:

Cilantro, stems and leaves, chopped (reserve 2 tbsp. leaves)	1 cup	Turmeric	1/4 tsp.
Garlic, minced	1 tsp.	Hawaiian chili, seeded and minced (optional)	1 small chili
Ginger, fresh, chopped fine	2 tbsp.	Kaffir lime leaves	2 each
Lemongrass, trimmed of outer stalks and chopped fine	3 stalks	Honey	1 tbsp.
Coconut milk, canned	1 cup	Hawaiian salt	1/4 tsp.
Curry powder	1 tbsp.	Reserve cooked carrot	2 chunks

1. Press and dry tofu, cut into slabs.
2. Cover a baking sheet or dish with canola oil and lay tofu slabs on the sheet; sprinkle with turmeric, curry powder and salt. Bake at 350 degrees for 30 minutes. Cool and cut into large squares.
3. Meanwhile, steam onion, carrot, sweet potato and potato chunks until just cooked. Cool a bit. Reserve 2 carrot chunks. Blend sauce ingredients with cooked carrots in a blender until smooth.
4. Sauté steamed vegetables with the 1 tbsp. canola oil, about 5 minutes or until slightly browned and crispy.
5. Add in the tofu and sauce and simmer for about 5 minutes to allow flavors to develop. Adjust to taste. Just before serving, stir in the reserved cilantro.

Nutrition note: The nutritional facts in this recipe show a high level of saturated fat, which comes from the coconut milk. However, realize that the curry sauce is used to coat the ingredients, and not all of the sauce created is consumed, as long as you do not pour sauce over your tofu, vegetables or rice.

Nutrition Facts

Serving Size (404g)

Amount Per Serving

Calories 440   Calories from Fat 220

	% Daily Value*
Total Fat 25g	38%
Saturated Fat 12g	60%
Trans Fat 0g	
Cholesterol 0mg	0%
Sodium 390mg	16%
Total Carbohydrate 44g	15%
Dietary Fiber 8g	32%
Sugars 13g	
Protein 17g	

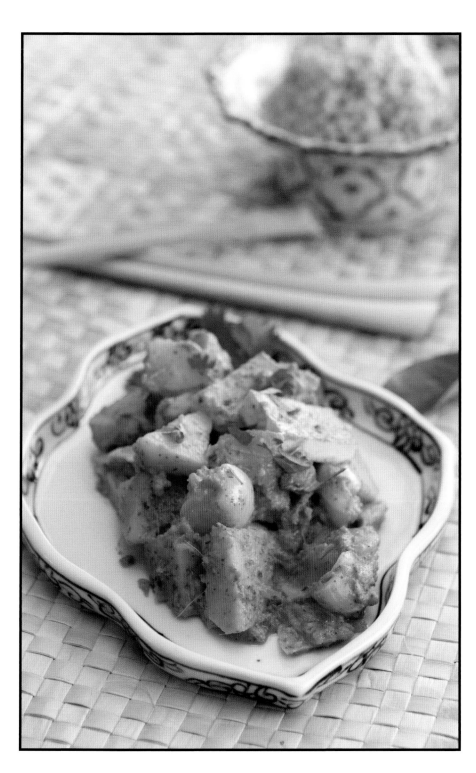

Steamed Sweet Potato and Swiss Chard Dumplings

By: Sharon Kobayashi

4 servings

Vegetable oil	1 tsp.
Garlic, minced	4 cloves
Sweet potato, minced	8 oz.
Swiss chard, finely sliced	8 oz.
Chinese 5-spice	1/2 tsp.
Mandoo (pot sticker) wrappers	20 each
Napa cabbage leaves	4 each
Basic Asian Vinaigrette (see below)	3 tbsp.
Water	1 tbsp.

Basic Asian Vinaigrette:

Shallot, minced (about 1/2 oz.)	1 tbsp.
Balsamic vinegar	2 tbsp.
Ginger, fresh, grated	1/2 tsp.
Sesame oil	1 tsp.
Soy sauce	1 tbsp.
Black pepper	to taste

1. Pre-heat a skillet over medium-high heat. Add oil, garlic and potato, and then sauté briefly for about 2 minutes.
2. Add Swiss chard and cook until all liquid from chard evaporates.
3. Remove from heat; add Chinese 5-spice. Cool thoroughly.
4. Lay out wrappers in a single layer. Distribute filling evenly, placing in the center of each wrapper.
5. Dip your finger in a bowl of water and trace edge of each wrapper. Don't get wrapper too wet.
6. Fold over and firmly press edges together to seal. Repeat until filling is used up.
7. Lay Napa cabbage leaves on bottom of steamer. Place dumplings over the leaves.
8. Steam until tender, approximately 15 minutes. Serve immediately.
9. Add water to vinaigrette. Serve 1 tbsp. sauce per person.

Tip: Dumplings can be frozen in a single layer. When completely frozen, transfer to a Ziplock bag. Do not defrost before using. The dumplings can also be cooked in boiling water: Bring water to a boil, add dumplings and reduce to medium heat. Cook for approximately 5 minutes.

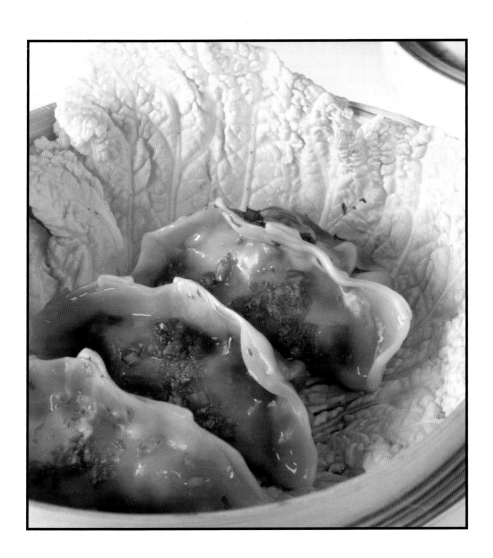

Nutrition Facts

Serving Size (200g)

Amount Per Serving

Calories 210   Calories from Fat 25

% Daily Value*

Total Fat 2.5g	**4%**
Saturated Fat 0g	**0%**
Trans Fat 0g	
Cholesterol 5mg	**2%**
Sodium 470mg	**20%**
Total Carbohydrate 40g	**13%**
Dietary Fiber 4g	**16%**
Sugars 5g	
Protein 7g	

3 to 4 servings

Simmered

Tofu, firm, (preferably Mrs. Cheng's), rinsed, drained and patted dry	1-20 oz. block
Salt (for simmering the tofu in water)	1 to 2 tsp.
Star anise, whole	4 each
Ginger, crushed	1 small piece

Sauce:

Light oil (safflower, or canola)	1 tbsp.
Salt	1/8 tsp.
Ginger, fresh, minced	2 tbsp.
Garlic, minced	1/2 tsp.
Green onions, minced	1/4 cup
Chinese parsley, minced	1/4 cup
Toasted sesame oil (optional)	1 tsp.

1. Cut tofu in half horizontally, then each half into 4 equal pieces.
2. In a pot of boiling water (use just enough to cover the tofu), add 1 to 2 tsp. salt, star anise and ginger.
3. Immerse the tofu and simmer for about 10 minutes.
4. Cool in broth, if possible.
5. Drain the tofu, pat dry and chill.
6. Heat oil and salt in a pan, then add the minced ginger, garlic, green onions, Chinese parsley.
7. Use a blender or food processor to combine the ingredients to a pesto-like in consistency (add 1 to 2 tbsp. water or additional oil if too thick.)
8. Cool and top tofu slices with a layer of the paste.

Tip: If you want to use even less oil, you can blend the minced ginger, garlic, green onions and Chinese parsley in the blender without heating them with the oil in Step 6.

Recipe continues on next page.

Pan-Fried

1. In a small sauté pan heat oil (macadamia nut, or high-oleic safflower, or non-GMO canola) oil with the star anise and ginger in medium heat for a few minutes to release the flavors.
2. Pan-fry the firm tofu slices lightly with the star anise-infused oil.
3. Top tofu with the ginger-green onion sauce.
4. It can be served either chilled or warm, with a side of brown rice.

Tip: A vegetarian's desire to re-create the flavors of the popular Chinese dish "Cold Ginger Chicken" is the motivation behind this recipe. If your tofu is not firm, you can wrap it in paper towels and place a firm weight on top to drain out excess fluid. Allow at least 15 minutes for this.

Nutrition note: The nutrition facts on this course show a slightly high reading on sodium (670g). The value accounts for all the sodium used in the recipe; however, the 1 to 2 tsp. salt is dissolved in the water to season the tofu while it is simmering. Not all of that salt will be added to the tofu once it is taken out of the liquid.

Nutrition Facts	
Serving Size (132g)	
Amount Per Serving	
Calories 160	Calories from Fat 110
	% Daily Value*
Total Fat 12g	**18%**
Saturated Fat 1.5g	**8%**
Trans Fat 0g	
Cholesterol 0mg	**0%**
Sodium 670mg	**28%**
Total Carbohydrate 3g	**1%**
Dietary Fiber 2g	**8%**
Sugars 0g	
Protein 13g	

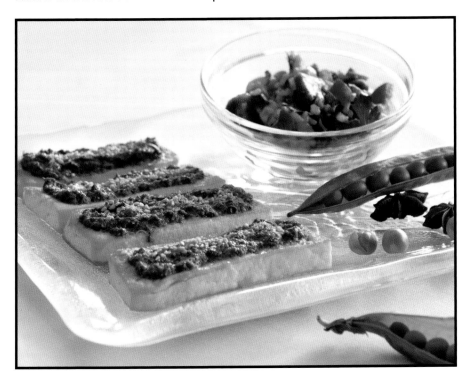

4 servings

Topping:

Moloka'i sweet potatoes	1 1/2 cups (about 2 each)
Yukon gold potatoes	1 1/2 cups (about 2 each)
Mustard	1 tsp.
Prepared horseradish	1/2 to 1 tsp.
Potato cooking water	as needed
Cheddar cheese, reduced-fat, grated (optional)	1/3 cup

1. Cook potatoes.
2. Mash with rest of ingredients, using the cooking water to desired consistency.

Filling:

Olive oil	1 tbsp.	Paprika	1/2 tsp.
Sweet Maui onion	1/2 cup	Hāmākua tomatoes, chopped	1 cup
Celery, chopped	1/2 cup	Tomato paste	1 tbsp.
Carrot, chopped	1/2 cup	Vegetable broth, low-sodium	
Garlic, minced	2 tsp.	(Pacific Foods or Imagine)	1/2 cup
Corn, fresh Kahuku (remove from		Vegetable Worcestershire	1 tsp.
the cob)	1 cup	Salt	1/4 tsp.
Mushrooms, fresh, sliced	1/2 cup	Pepper	1/2 tsp.
Vegetarian meat (soy beef, Yves		Flour	1 tbsp.
Good Ground Veggie Original)	1 cup	Water	2 tbsp.
Oregano	1/2 tsp.		

1. Heat oil in a large skillet.
2. Sauté onions, celery and carrot for about 5 minutes or until they begin to soften.
3. Add in the garlic, corn, mushrooms and sauté a few minutes more.
4. Next, add in the soy "beef," oregano and paprika; cook two minutes.
5. Mix flour and water to make a slurry. Add in the tomatoes, tomato paste, broth, Worcestershire, salt, pepper and slurry. Cook until the sauce thickens.
6. Pour into a prepared 9" pie plate or 8"x8" baking dish and top with mashed potato mixture.
7. Bake at 350 degrees for about 25 to 30 minutes or until hot and bubbly.

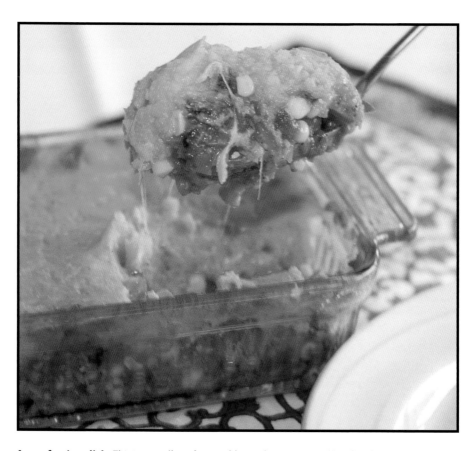

A comforting dish: This is a medley of vegetables and a soy "ground beef" substitute stir fried, seasoned with savory herbs and then simmered in a tomato-based sauce. This is then topped with a flavorful combination of local sweet potato mashed with Yukon gold, mustard and low-fat cheddar cheese. Baked just enough to heat through, all this dish needs is a green salad to make a complete meal.

Substitutions: White potato can be used instead of Yukon gold. Any veggie burger or soy-crumbles can be used if you cannot find Yves soy-ground (note that the sodium levels may differ). Water can be used instead of broth. Regular Worcestershire can be interchanged with the vegetarian version.

Nutrition Facts

Serving Size (483g)

Amount Per Serving

Calories 380	Calories from Fat 60

	% Daily Value*
Total Fat 7g	11%
Saturated Fat 2g	10%
Trans Fat 0g	
Cholesterol 5mg	2%
Sodium 560mg	23%
Total Carbohydrate 64g	21%
Dietary Fiber 11g	44%
Sugars 10g	
Protein 17g	

Vegetable Curry Pita
By: Sharon Kobayashi

8 servings

Vegetable oil	1 tbsp.	Cabbage, shredded	4 oz.
Onion, 1/4" dice	1 each (about 10 oz.)	Salt	1/2 tsp.
Garlic, minced	6 cloves	Soy sauce	1 tsp.
Curry powder	1 tbsp.	Peanut butter	1/4 cup
Tomato, 1/4" dice	1 each (about 6 oz.)	Lemon juice	1 to 2 tsp.
Cauliflower, 1/4" dice	1 lb.	Cilantro, fresh	to taste
Bell pepper, 1/4" dice	1 each (about 7 oz.)	Pita bread	8 halves

1. Sauté onion in oil until deep brown.
2. Add garlic and curry powder. Sauté briefly.
3. Add vegetables and salt. Cover and cook until tender, about 10 minutes.
4. Very little liquid should be left in the pan. If too wet, continue to cook uncovered.
5. Remove from heat and stir in peanut butter, lemon juice and cilantro.
6. Cool completely in the refrigerator.

Tip: Freeze unused portions for later use. Filling is also good wrapped in a tortilla. The sodium content of this dish comes mainly from the pita bread. If that is a concern, add this dish to rice or rice noodles.

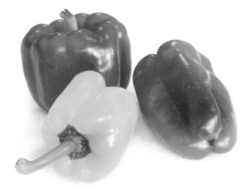

Nutrition Facts
Serving Size (206g)

Amount Per Serving

Calories 270　　　Calories from Fat 60

	% Daily Value*
Total Fat 7g	**11%**
Saturated Fat 1g	**5%**
Trans Fat 0g	
Cholesterol 0mg	**0%**
Sodium 560mg	**23%**
Total Carbohydrate 47g	**16%**
Dietary Fiber 8g	**32%**
Sugars 5g	
Protein 11g	

Asian-Style Lettuce Wraps

By: Alyssa Moreau

4 servings

Sauce:

Rice vinegar	1 tbsp.	Sugar	1 tsp.
Soy sauce, low-sodium	1 tbsp.	Pepper	1/4 tsp.
Sambal chile paste	1/4 tsp.	Tofu, fresh firm, cut into 1/2-inch pieces	1/2 block

Main Dish:

Oil	1 tbsp.
Ginger, fresh, minced	1 tbsp.
Garlic, minced	1 large clove
Shiitake mushrooms, fresh, sliced	1/2 cup
Boca burgers cut into cubes, or soy "ground beef"	2 burgers
Water chestnuts, chopped	1 small can
Green onions, sliced, 1 tbsp. reserved for garnish	1/2 cup
Roma tomato, seeded and chopped fine	1 each
Sesame seeds, toasted	1 tbsp.
Lettuce, rinsed and dried (such as Mānoa)	12 leaves
Brown rice, cooked	2 to 3 cups

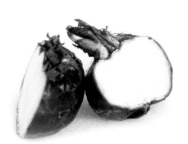

1. In a large bowl, combine sauce ingredients, except tofu.
2. Add the tofu and lightly toss to coat the tofu. Let sit and marinate while preparing the rest of the dish.
3. Add oil to skillet and sauté the ginger, garlic and mushrooms for a few minutes.
4. When the mushrooms start to soften, add the soy "beef" and continue to stir-fry until lightly browned.
5. Add back in the tofu-marinade mixture. Add the water chestnuts and green onions (minus 1 tbsp. reserved for garnish). Cook for a few minutes then transfer to a serving plate.
6. To garnish, top with tomato pieces, sesame seeds and reserved green onions.
7. Serve in lettuce leaves with brown rice.

Nutrition Facts

Serving Size (324g)

Amount Per Serving

Calories 340   Calories from Fat 90

	% Daily Value*
Total Fat 10g	**15%**
Saturated Fat 1g	**5%**
Trans Fat 0g	
Cholesterol 0mg	**0%**
Sodium 250mg	**10%**
Total Carbohydrate 50g	**17%**
Dietary Fiber 8g	**32%**
Sugars 4g	
Protein 17g	

8 servings

Shiso leaves, minced	10 each
Shallot, minced	1 each (approximately 2 tbsp.)
Pine nuts, toasted and minced	1 tbsp.
Soy sauce	2 tsp.
Lemon juice	2 tbsp.
Lemon zest	1/4 tsp.
Ume (Asian plum), paste	1 tsp.
Spinach, minced	1 oz. (approximately 2 tbsp.)
Dijon mustard	1 tsp.
Extra-virgin olive oil	3 tbsp.

1. Combine all ingredients and pulse in a food processor.
2. Let pesto rest approximately 1 hour and refrigerate before using.

Fish:

4 servings

Fish, mild, firm (ʻōpakapaka or opah)	1 lb.

1. Marinate 4 oz. mild, firm-fleshed fresh fish per person in 1 tsp. pesto each.
2. Marinate for approximately 10 minutes.
3. In a hot skillet, cook fish until browned and cooked through, about 6 to 7 minutes.
4. Serve fish topped with an additional 2 tsp. pesto.

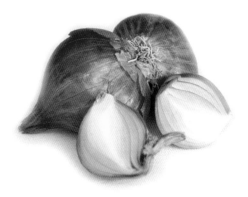

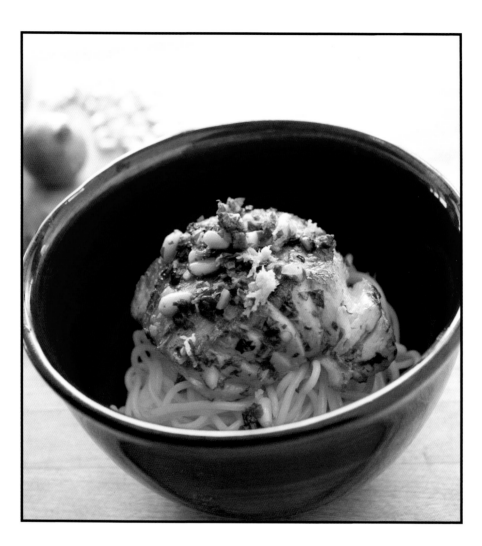

Nutrition Facts

Serving Size (134g)

Amount Per Serving

Calories 190   Calories from Fat 80

	% Daily Value*
Total Fat 9g	**14**%
Saturated Fat 1.5g	**8**%
Trans Fat 0g	
Cholesterol 40mg	**13**%
Sodium 130mg	**5**%
Total Carbohydrate 2g	**1**%
Dietary Fiber 0g	**0**%
Sugars 0g	
Protein 24g	

Cucumber Bisque with Cherry Tomato Garnish   By: Alyssa Moreau

4 servings

Soup:

Japanese cucumbers, large, peeled and seeded, chopped in large chunks	4 each (8 cups)
Cilantro, chopped	1/2 cup
Green onions, chopped	1/4 cup
Plain yogurt, low-fat	2 cups
Olive oil	1 tbsp.
Lime juice, fresh	2 tbsp.
Salt	1/2 tsp.
Black pepper	1/4 tsp.

Garnish:

Cherry tomatoes, sliced in halves or quarters	2 cups
Olive oil	4 tsp.
Cilantro, chopped	4 tsp.
Green onions, sliced	4 tsp.
Black pepper, cracked/fresh ground	1 tsp.

Combine the ingredients for the soup in a blender and blend until smooth. Adjust flavors to taste. Pour into individual serving bowls and garnish with the cherry tomatoes, a drizzle of olive oil, cilantro and green onions. Grind some fresh pepper, if desired.

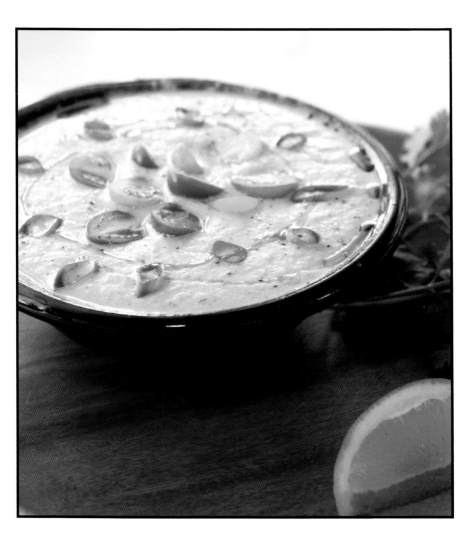

Nutrition Facts

Serving Size (436g)

Amount Per Serving

Calories 190   Calories from Fat 90

% Daily Value*

Total Fat 10g	**15%**
Saturated Fat 2.5g	**13%**
Trans Fat 0g	
Cholesterol 10mg	**3%**
Sodium 380mg	**16%**
Total Carbohydrate 17g	**6%**
Dietary Fiber 4g	**16%**
Sugars 12g	
Protein 9g	

Curried Sweet Potato Chowder

By: Alyssa Moreau

4 servings

Butter or margarine	1 tbsp.		Soymilk	3 cups, or as needed
Shallot (2 to 3 large), minced	1/2 cup		Peas, frozen	2 cups
Curry powder	1 1/2 tsp.		Pumpkin seeds, curried*	1/2 cup
Sweet potatoes, cubed	1 3/4 lbs. (about 3 cups)		Cilantro, chopped	1/2 cup
Vegetable broth	4 cups		Salt and pepper	to taste

1. Melt the butter in a large saucepan. Add shallots and cook for 2 to 3 minutes. Sprinkle in the curry powder, stir for about 30 seconds.
2. Add sweet potato and broth. Cover and simmer for 20 minutes or until sweet potato is tender. Let cool; then transfer to a blender, add the soymilk to cover and blend until smooth. Add more milk if it is too thick.
3. Transfer back to saucepan and add the peas. Cook a few minutes or until the peas are heated through.
4. Add salt and pepper to taste.
5. Serve in individual bowls topped with the curried pumpkin seeds and chopped cilantro.

*To make curried pumpkin seeds: sauté pumpkin seeds in a bit of olive oil; sprinkle with curry powder and a dash of cayenne and salt. Remove from the heat when they start to pop.

Nutrition Facts

Serving Size (736g)

Amount Per Serving

Calories 500   Calories from Fat 150

	% Daily Value*
Total Fat 17g	**26%**
Saturated Fat 2.5g	**13%**
Trans Fat 0g	
Cholesterol 0mg	**0%**
Sodium 390mg	**16%**
Total Carbohydrate 68g	**23%**
Dietary Fiber 14g	**56%**
Sugars 15g	
Protein 21g	

Green Tea and Rice "Soup" with Baby Shanghai Cabbage

4 servings

By: Alyssa Moreau

Green tea leaves or 2 teabags	2 tsp.
Water	2 cups
Sesame oil	1 tbsp.
Sweet Maui onion, sliced into 1/2-moons	1/2 cup
Shiitake mushrooms, fresh, sliced	1/2 cup

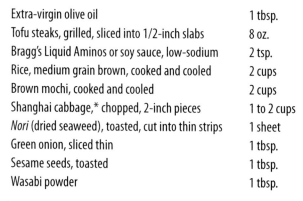

Extra-virgin olive oil	1 tbsp.
Tofu steaks, grilled, sliced into 1/2-inch slabs	8 oz.
Bragg's Liquid Aminos or soy sauce, low-sodium	2 tsp.
Rice, medium grain brown, cooked and cooled	2 cups
Brown mochi, cooked and cooled	2 cups
Shanghai cabbage,* chopped, 2-inch pieces	1 to 2 cups
Nori (dried seaweed), toasted, cut into thin strips	1 sheet
Green onion, sliced thin	1 tbsp.
Sesame seeds, toasted	1 tbsp.
Wasabi powder	1 tbsp.

1. Bring water to a boil and brew tea for about 2 minutes. Take out tea leaves or bags, set aside.
2. Sauté the onions and shiitake in sesame oil until translucent and soft.
3. Sauté the tofu steaks in olive oil until crisp and brown. Pour Bragg's or low-sodium soy sauce over steaks as they finish cooking.
4. Place rice and mochi in four deep bowls, topping the onion/shiitake mixture, then with the Shanghai cabbage and lastly the tofu steaks. Pour hot brewed tea into bowls until rice is nearly submerged.
5. Garnish the bowls of tofu and rice with the nori, green onion and toasted sesame seeds.
6. In a small bowl, dilute the wasabi with some of the same tea. Serve on the side.

*Shanghai cabbage is often misnamed "baby bok choy." It has slightly curved, spoon-shaped green stems, whereas bok choy is a white-stemmed cabbage with dark green leaves. Both come in the large forms and the smaller "baby" versions, which are less bitter and have a brighter flavor.

Nutrition Facts

Serving Size (677g)

Amount Per Serving

Calories 390	Calories from Fat 100	
		% Daily Value*
Total Fat 11g		**17%**
Saturated Fat 1.5g		**8%**
Trans Fat 0g		
Cholesterol 0mg		**0%**
Sodium 190mg		**8%**
Total Carbohydrate 60g		**20%**
Dietary Fiber 3g		**12%**
Sugars 2g		
Protein 13g		

Moloka'i Sweet Potato-Lemongrass Bisque By: Alyssa Moreau

4 servings

Olive oil	1 tbsp.
Sweet onion, chopped	1 cup
Garlic, minced	1 tsp.
Ginger, fresh, minced	1 tbsp.
Moloka'i sweet potato, peeled and chopped	2 lbs. (about 6 cups)
Carrot, chopped	1 cup
Lemongrass, outer layers and green leaves removed, bulbs split open	3 stalks
Kaffir lime leaves,* torn	2 leaves
Vegetable broth, low-sodium	2 cups
Coconut milk, canned	1/4 cup
Salt	1/2 tsp.
Cayenne pepper	dash
Cilantro leaves, chopped	2 tbsp.

1. Heat olive oil in a pot and add onion. Cook about 5 minutes, until soft.
2. Add garlic, ginger and cook 1 minute.
3. Add the sweet potatoes, carrot, lemongrass and kaffir lime leaves (or 1 tbsp. fresh lime juice).
4. Add broth and enough water to cover contents and bring to a boil.
5. Reduce heat to medium, cover and simmer until potatoes are tender, about 15 to 20 minutes.
6. Remove lemongrass and kaffir lime leaves.
7. Reserve 1 1/2 cups cooking liquid then add the coconut milk, salt and cayenne pepper.
8. Blend in a blender until smooth. (Add lime juice at this time if not using kaffir lime leaves.*)
9. Add more water if too thick to create desired consistency.
10. Garnish with the cilantro.

*This soup is seasoned with fresh lemongrass, kaffir lime leaves and a bit of coconut milk to enhance the flavor. Kaffir lime leaves and lemongrass are common ingredients used in Southeast Asian cookery and can be found at the local farmers markets as well as some grocery stores. They are fibrous and are not for ingestion, but they are very aromatic, adding a refreshing fragrance to the dish. You can substitute fresh lime juice for the kaffir lime leaves (1 tbsp. juice, to taste).

The ginger can also be substituted with galangal, also known as Thai ginger, which imparts an additional aromatic dimension to the soup. All these ingredients are found at farmers markets and Chinatown markets in downtown Honolulu.

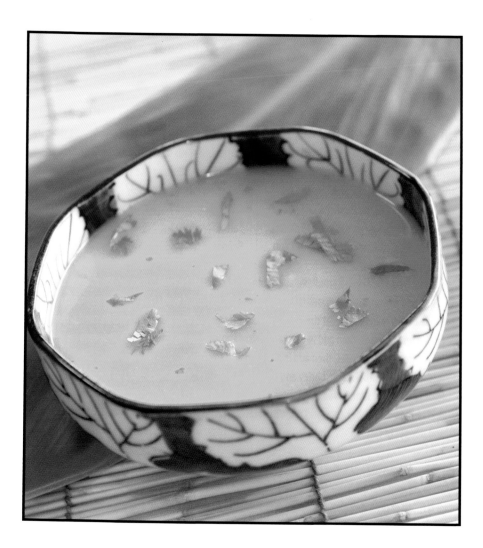

Nutrition Facts

Serving Size (441g)

Amount Per Serving

Calories 290   Calories from Fat 60

% Daily Value*

Total Fat 7g	**11**%
Saturated Fat 3g	**15**%
Trans Fat 0g	
Cholesterol 0mg	**0**%
Sodium 440mg	**18**%
Total Carbohydrate 54g	**18**%
Dietary Fiber 9g	**36**%
Sugars 14g	
Protein 5g	

Miso Saimin with Shanghai Cabbage

By: Sharon Kobyashi

2 servings

Saimin, 4.5 oz. each, frozen, without soup base	2 packages
Japanese stock (see recipe on page 136)	2 cups
Baby bok choy (Shanghai cabbage)	8 oz.
Daikon, peel and julienne	2 oz.
Miso, white, mixed with 2 tbsp. cold water until dissolved	1 tbsp.
Green onions, sliced	to taste

1. Cook saimin according to package directions. Do not use soup base. Strain.
2. Bring stock to boil, add cabbage and daikon and cook until tender, about 2 minutes.
3. Add noodles, miso and green onions, and then remove from heat and serve.

Serving suggestion: Add grated ginger, minced garlic, fresh basil, cilantro, mint and sliced hot peppers.

Festive Gazpacho

By: Alyssa Moreau

2 servings

Tomato juice, low-sodium	1 1/2 cups	Olive oil	2 tbsp
Tomato, fresh, diced	2 cups	Red wine or balsamic vinegar	2 tbsp.
Cucumber, peeled and seeded,		Lime juice	2 tbsp.
cut into chunks	2 cups	Worcestershire sauce	1/4 to 1/2 tsp.
Red bell pepper, chopped	1/2 cup	Hot sauce	1/2 tsp.
Garlic, minced	1 tsp.	Cracked pepper	1/8 tsp.

Garnish:

Avocado, cut into chunks	1/4 to 1/2 cup
Green onions, sliced thin	2 tbsp.
Paprika to sprinkle over	1 tsp.
Olive oil to drizzle	1 tsp.

1. Combine all the ingredients except the garnish and blend to desired consistency.
2. Garnish with avocado and green onions.
3. Sprinkle with paprika and drizzle with a bit of olive oil.

Nutrition Facts

Serving Size (611g)

Amount Per Serving

Calories 290   Calories from Fat 180

	% Daily Value*
Total Fat 20g	31%
Saturated Fat 3g	15%
Trans Fat 0g	
Cholesterol 0mg	0%
Sodium 135mg	6%
Total Carbohydrate 24g	8%
Dietary Fiber 6g	24%
Sugars 15g	
Protein 5g	

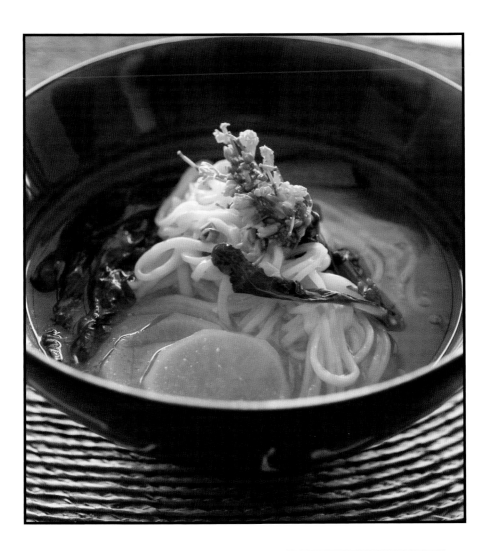

Nutrition Facts

Serving Size (571g)

Amount Per Serving

Calories 260   Calories from Fat 10

% Daily Value*

Total Fat 1.5g	**2%**
Saturated Fat 0g	**0%**
Trans Fat 0g	
Cholesterol 5mg	**2%**
Sodium 420mg	**18%**
Total Carbohydrate 50g	**17%**
Dietary Fiber 8g	**32%**
Sugars 3g	
Protein 14g	

Chicken Adobo Wilted Salad

By: Sharon Kobayashi

6 servings

Chicken thighs, boneless, skinless and cut into bite size	8 oz.
Chicken tenders, 99% fat-free, cut into bite-size pieces	8 oz.
Garbanzo beans, rinsed and drained	1 can
Garlic, sliced thin	6 cloves
Mushrooms, halved	4 oz.
Balsamic vinegar, plus extra for seasoning	1/2 cup
Soy sauce	1 tsp.
Bay leaves	4 leaves
Peppercorns	10 each
Chicken broth, reduced-sodium	2/3 cup
Extra-virgin olive oil	1 tbsp.
Baby arugula	6 cups

1. Add all ingredients (except chicken broth, olive oil and arugula) in a pot with a cover.
2. Bring to a boil, reduce to medium heat.
3. Cook, partially covered, until liquids are evaporated in about 10 minutes.
4. Add chicken broth, scraping the bottom of pot.
5. Remove from heat. Add olive oil and more vinegar, if desired.
6. Top salad greens with hot chicken mix and toss to combine.
7. Serve immediately with crusty rolls.

Substitutions: The baby arugula can be replaced with baby *tatsoi* (spinach mustard greens) or baby spinach for a milder flavor. For a spicier salad, slightly crush the peppercorns. Use steamed watercress or choy sum if cooked vegetables are preferred, and serve with brown rice.

Nutrition Facts

Serving Size (275g)

Amount Per Serving

Calories 210	Calories from Fat 50
	% Daily Value*
Total Fat 6g	9%
Saturated Fat 1g	5%
Trans Fat 0g	
Cholesterol 55mg	18%
Sodium 180mg	8%
Total Carbohydrate 19g	6%
Dietary Fiber 5g	20%
Sugars 6g	
Protein 22g	

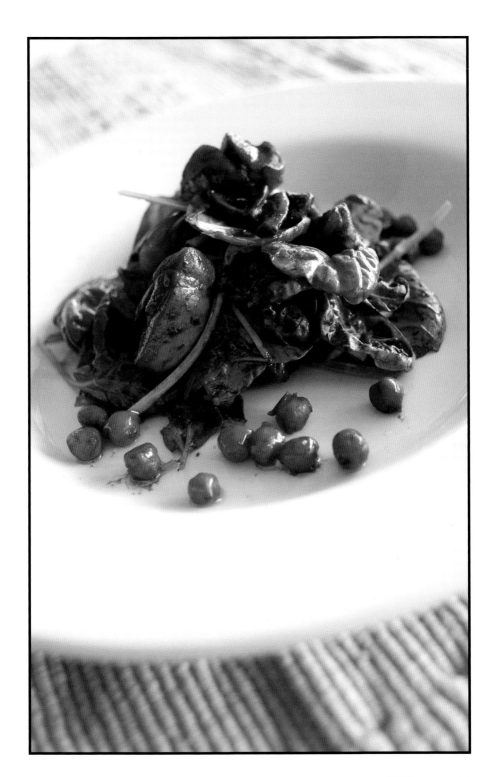

Cucumber Salad with Japanese-Flavored Dressing By: Alyssa Moreau

3 servings

Japanese cucumbers, seeded and thinly sliced into half-moons	3 cups
Rice vinegar	1/4 cup
Wasabi powder	1/2 to 1 tsp.
Sugar	2 tsp.
Soy sauce, low-salt	1 tbsp.
Pickled ginger, minced	2 to 3 tsp.
Furikake (with nori seaweed and sesame seeds)	1/2 tsp.

Nutrition Facts

Serving Size (163g)

Amount Per Serving

Calories 40	Calories from Fat 0

	% Daily Value*
Total Fat 0g	0%
Saturated Fat 0g	0%
Trans Fat 0g	
Cholesterol 0mg	0%
Sodium 230mg	10%
Total Carbohydrate 8g	3%
Dietary Fiber 2g	8%
Sugars 5g	
Protein 2g	

1. Place cucumbers in a large bowl.
2. In a smaller bowl, stir together the vinegar, wasabi powder, sugar and soy sauce. Stir into cucumbers. Garnish with furikake.

Hawaiian Waldorf Salad

4 servings

Jicama (chop suey yam), diced 1/2-inch	2 cups	Black pepper, ground fresh	to taste
Celery stalks, diced 1/2-inch	3 each	Macadamia nut pieces, toasted and cooled	4 tbsp.
Smoked turkey breast, diced 1/2-inch	8 oz.	Mānoa lettuce, leaves only, washed and dried	1 head
Raisins	1/3 cup		
Papaya, ripe but firm, diced 1-inch	1/2 each		
Mayonnaise, low-fat	1/4 cup		
Onion, minced and squeezed dry	1 tbsp.		
Tarragon, fresh, minced	1 tsp.		
Lemon, juice and zest of 1 lemon	2 Tbsp.		
Dijon mustard	1 tsp.		

Nutrition Facts

Serving Size (297g)

Amount Per Serving

Calories 260	Calories from Fat 110

	% Daily Value*
Total Fat 12g	18%
Saturated Fat 2g	10%
Trans Fat 0g	
Cholesterol 25mg	8%
Sodium 750mg	31%
Total Carbohydrate 28g	9%
Dietary Fiber 7g	28%
Sugars 15g	
Protein 12g	

1. Combine first 5 ingredients in a bowl.
2. In another bowl, mix together mayonnaise, onion, tarragon, lime juice and zest, mustard and pepper.
3. Gently toss dressing and salad together until coated.
4. Divide lettuce onto 4 plates, and garnish with 1 tbsp. macadamia nuts, and an extra grinding of pepper.

Edamame, Tomato, Hawaiian Corn and Artichoke Salad

By: Alyssa Moreau

4 servings

Edamame (soybeans), fresh or frozen soybeans, shelled	2 cups
Tomatoes, fresh, seeded and chopped	2 cups
Corn, fresh, sliced off the cob	2 cups
Red bell pepper, chopped fine	1 each
Marinated artichoke hearts, drained and chopped (liquid reserved)	1-6 oz. jar
Sweet Maui onion, minced	2 tbsp.
Cilantro, fresh, chopped	1/4 cup

Dressing:

Silken tofu (preferably soft)	6 oz.
Rice vinegar	2 tbsp.
Prepared mustard (stoneground or Dijon-style)	1 tbsp.
Salt	1/4 tsp.
Pepper	1/4 tsp.
Basil or parsley, fresh, julienne	1 tbsp.
Mānoa or green-leaf lettuce	4 cups

1. Bring a large pot of water to a boil.
2. Add beans and cook for about 8 minutes or until beans are done. Drain well.
3. In a salad bowl, combine beans, tomato, corn, bell pepper, artichokes, onion and cilantro.
4. In a blender or food processor, combine tofu, vinegar, artichoke liquid,* mustard, salt and pepper.
5. Process until smooth and pour over vegetables. Add the basil and toss to mix well. Serve on bed of lettuce.

* or 2 tbsp. olive oil and 1 tbsp. water

Nutrition Facts

Serving Size (409g)

Amount Per Serving

Calories 220   Calories from Fat 70

	% Daily Value*
Total Fat 8g	**12%**
Saturated Fat 0g	**0%**
Trans Fat 0g	
Cholesterol 0mg	**0%**
Sodium 370mg	**15%**
Total Carbohydrate 32g	**11%**
Dietary Fiber 10g	**40%**
Sugars 9g	
Protein 13g	

3 to 4 servings

Black Japonica rice* (plus 2 cups water)	1 cup	Carrot, 1/4" diced	1/2 cup
Brown mochi rice or pearl barley		Red bell pepper, chopped	1/2 cup
(plus 1 cup water)	1/2 cup	Italian parsley, flat leaf, chopped	1/4 cup
Wild rice (plus 2 cups water)	1 cup	Olive oil	1 to 2 tbsp.
Beans, great northern, low- or no-salt		Salt	1/4 to 1/2 tsp.
canned, rinsed and drained	1 cup	Pepper	dash
Peas, defrosted	1 cup	Mānoa lettuce	one head
Okinawan sweet potato, cubed, cooked	1 cup		

*A very high quality black Japonica rice is distributed by Lotus Foods under the registered trademark name "Forbidden Black Rice." It is used in Chinese and Southeast Asian savory dishes and deserts. This rice bleeds beet-red when you rinse it, and once cooked it ends up a striking deep burgundy. It holds its shape very well and is pleasantly chewy. With a subtle sweetness and a rich taste, it adds a striking appearance to the dish. A blend of all three rices is available at health food stores.

Tip: 1 cup dry Japonica rice and 1 3/4 cups water produces 3 3/4 cups cooked rice.
Cooking time: 35 minutes

1. Cook grains separately. Drain if necessary.
2. Combine rest of ingredients with grains and add olive oil, salt and pepper to taste.
3. Serve on a bed of Mānoa lettuce.

A colorful dish that is great to take as a potluck dish to parties. The rice blend used can also be found at any local health food store. The wild rice adds a textured variance with a nice bite, and the Okinawan sweet potatoes add a wonderful color and natural sweetness, rounding out the other added flavors of the vegetables that make up this dish. Feel free to substitute with other vegetables, such as sweet onion, celery, corn, diced zucchini and cilantro, to create variations.

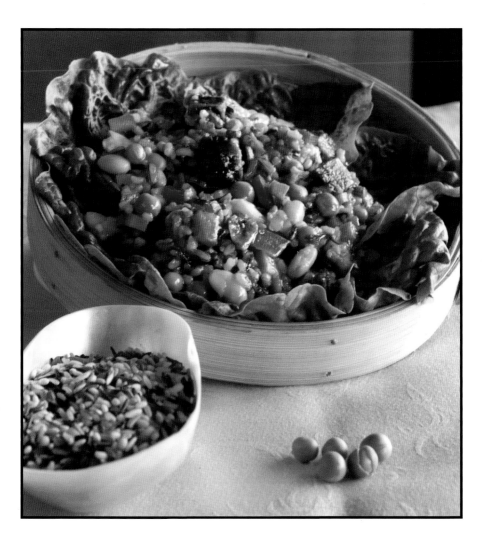

Nutrition Facts		
Serving Size (409g)		

Amount Per Serving

Calories 590	Calories from Fat 90	
		% Daily Value*
Total Fat 10g		**15**%
Saturated Fat 1.5g		**8**%
Trans Fat 0g		
Cholesterol 0mg		**0**%
Sodium 400mg		**17**%
Total Carbohydrate 111g		**37**%
Dietary Fiber 15g		**60**%
Sugars 7g		
Protein 18g		

4 servings

Kahuku corn, fresh, with kernels cut off	4 ears (4 cups)
Hāmākua tomatoes, ripe, chopped	2 cups
Black olives, cut in half	1/4 cup
Sweet Maui onion, thinly sliced slivers	1/4 cup
Basil, fresh, julienne	1/2 cup
Garlic clove, pressed	1 tsp.
Extra-virgin olive oil	2 tbsp.
White balsamic or rice vinegar	1 tbsp.
Salt	1/4 tsp.
Pepper	1/8 tsp.
Mānoa or green-leaf lettuce	2 cups

Toss all together in a large bowl and let sit for about 1 hour to allow flavors to develop and absorb into the vegetables. Serve on bed of lettuce.

Tip: Fresh, locally-grown tomatoes are full of flavor and taste sweet and juicy, not watery like the tomatoes that are picked green and ripened in containers enroute to Hawai'i. Tomatoes are best kept in a cool place at room temperature, not refrigerated. This is a dish that allows for a great variation of texture and flavors depending on the type of olives (green, black, cured), tomatoes (red, yellow), onions (sweet, red) and salad greens (lettuce, spring greens, spinach) that you use.

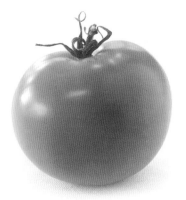

Nutrition Facts

Serving Size (309g)

Amount Per Serving

Calories 240	Calories from Fat 90

	% Daily Value*
Total Fat 10g	15%
Saturated Fat 1.5g	8%
Trans Fat 0g	
Cholesterol 0mg	0%
Sodium 250mg	10%
Total Carbohydrate 36g	12%
Dietary Fiber 6g	24%
Sugars 9g	
Protein 6g	

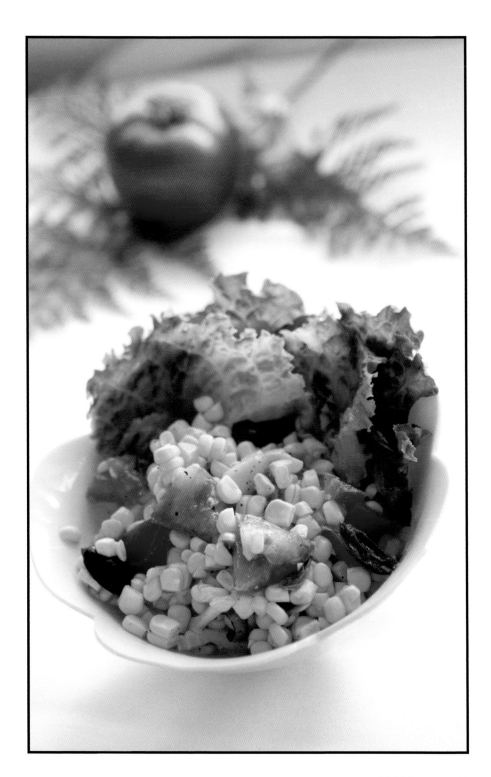

Salad with Okinawan Sweet Potato Crisps
By: Sharon Kobayashi

4 servings

Okinawan sweet potato, or other firm-fleshed sweet potato, boiled	1 lb.
Cream cheese, light	1 oz.
Milk, skim	1/2 cup
Phyllo dough	12 sheets
Almonds, sliced, toasted	1 oz. (4 tbsp.)
Cranberries, dried	2 oz. (1/2 cup)
Salad dressing (favorite vinaigrette style)	1/2 cup
Napa cabbage, shredded	8 cups

1. Mash sweet potato, stir in cream cheese and milk. Cool.
2. Pre-heat oven to 400 degrees. Spray a baking sheet with cooking spray.
3. Using 2 sheets of phyllo at a time, lay flat, spray with cooking spray.
4. Spread 1/3 cup cooked, mashed sweet potato in an even line along the edge of the longer side of the phyllo sheet.
5. Roll the phyllo sheet, starting from the side with the mashed sweet potato, tightly like a cigar. Cut in half. Transfer to baking sheet.
6. Repeat with remaining sheets of phyllo dough and potato.
7. Spray finished rolls with cooking spray.
8. Bake for 30 minutes or until brown. Cool on rack.
9. Toss almonds and cranberries with salad dressing and cabbage.
10. Serve immediately.

Tip: Keep phyllo covered with slightly damp paper towels to avoid drying out until needed. If not using within 2 weeks, wrap unused portion of dough well with plastic wrap and store in freezer.

Nutrition note: The nutrition facts reflect the sodium level for a typical vinaigrette dressing found at supermarkets. If you make your own vinaigrette, the sodium level would be much lower and you can add your own mixture of herbs and seasoning to create variations. See recipes in "Sides & Basics."

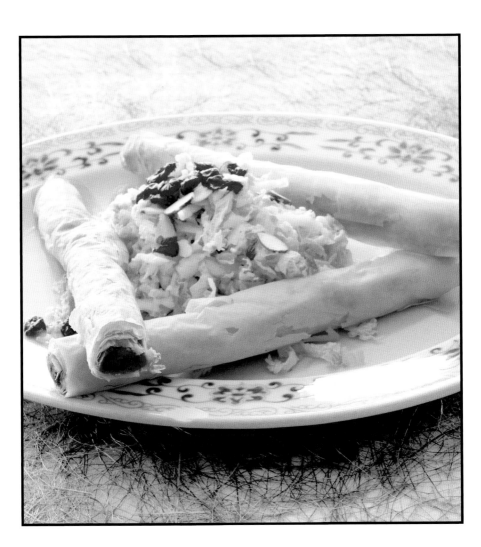

Nutrition Facts	
Serving Size (413g)	
Amount Per Serving	
Calories 500 Calories from Fat 150	
	% Daily Value*
Total Fat 16g	**25%**
Saturated Fat 3g	**15%**
Trans Fat 0g	
Cholesterol 5mg	**2%**
Sodium 710mg	**30%**
Total Carbohydrate 76g	**25%**
Dietary Fiber 8g	**32%**
Sugars 21g	
Protein 11g	

6 servings

Wild rice	4 oz. (about 3/4 cup)
Tomatoes, diced	2 each
Japanese cucumber, diced	1 each
Italian parsley, minced	2 bunch (about 3 oz.)
Mint, minced	1 bunch (about 1 1/2 oz.)
Onion, minced	2 tbsp.
Green onion	2 stalks
Feta cheese	1/2 cup
Extra-virgin olive oil	2 tbsp.
Lemon juice	2 tbsp. (about 1 lemon)
Lemon zest	1 lemon
Salt	1/4 tsp.
Pepper	to taste

1. Bring rice and about 4 cups of water to a boil, reduce to medium. Cook 45 to 50 minutes.
2. Drain rice well and cool.
3. Combine all other ingredients. Add rice and let rest, refrigerated 1 hour before serving.

Suggest serving with 1 serving of Edamame Imitation Guacamole spread on 1 pita bread.

Edamame Imitation "Guacamole"

6 servings

Soybeans, shelled	1 lb.
Frozen spinach, thawed	2 oz. (about 1/4 cup)
Cream cheese, light	2 oz. (about 1/4 cup)
Garlic	2 cloves
Sesame oil	1/2 tsp.
Cumin	1 tsp.
Salt	1/2 tsp.
Lemon juice	1 tbsp. (to taste)
Water	1/2 cup
Jalapeño, minced, seeds and veins removed	1 each
Cilantro, minced	to taste

1. Boil soybeans until very tender.
2. Add all ingredients to a food processor and process until very smooth.
3. Add more water if mixture is too thick.
4. Store covered, in the refrigerator.

Serving suggestion: This imitation guacamole is a perfect substitution if you are concerned about the cholesterol level in avocados. You can serve it as a sandwich with a whole-wheat pita bread, sliced cucumbers, tomato and baby arugula. You can also serve it as a dip alongside the wild rice tabouleh with pita wedges.

Nutrition Facts

Serving Size (153g)

Amount Per Serving

Calories 180	Calories from Fat 80

	% Daily Value*
Total Fat 8g	**12%**
Saturated Fat 2.5g	**13%**
Trans Fat 0g	
Cholesterol 10mg	**3%**
Sodium 280mg	**12%**
Total Carbohydrate 21g	**7%**
Dietary Fiber 3g	**12%**
Sugars 3g	
Protein 7g	

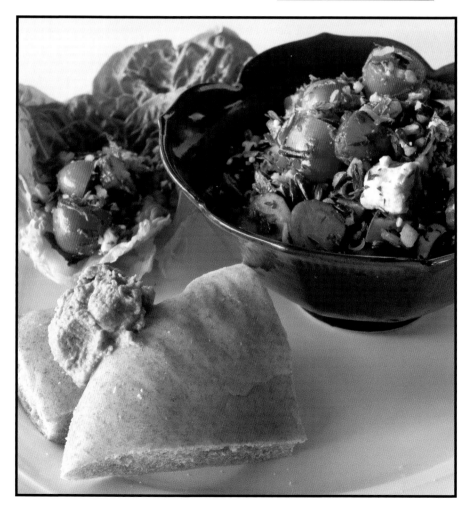

4 servings

Kabocha pumpkin, peeled, seeded and cut into 1-inch chunks	4 cups
Red bell pepper, sliced	1 cup
Leek, sliced thin	1 cup
Garlic, minced	2 tsp.
Olive oil	1 tbsp.
Cumin	1 tsp.
Salt	1/4 tsp.
Cayenne	dash
Beans, cannellini or great northern, low-sodium or salt-free, rinsed and drained	1-15 oz. can
Sesame seeds, toasted	1 tbsp.
Cilantro or parsley, chopped	1/4 cup
Mesclun greens	12 cups

Dressing:

Olive oil	3 tbsp.
White balsamic vinegar, or rice vinegar	3 tbsp.
Soy sauce, low-sodium	1 tbsp.
Hawaiian lehua honey or macadamia nut oil	1 tbsp.
Lime juice	1/2 lime

1. Toss together the kabocha, bell pepper, leek, garlic, olive oil, cumin, salt and cayenne until well mixed.
2. Place in a 9"x13" pan and bake at 350 degrees for 30 minutes or until the kabocha is cooked through.
3. Cool slightly, then add in the beans, sesame seeds and cilantro.
4. Combine dressing ingredients in a jar and shake well. Adjust flavors to taste.
5. Pour 1/2 over the pumpkin mixture and serve on bed of mesclun greens with extra dressing on the side.

Substitutions:
1. Butternut squash can be substituted for Kabocha pumpkin.
2. Any white beans can be used, such as navy or garbanzo beans.
3. Agave nectar can be used in place of honey.

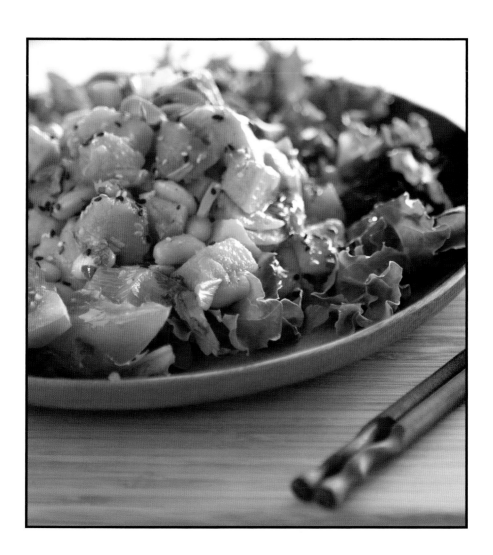

Nutrition Facts

Serving Size (478g)

Amount Per Serving

Calories 340   Calories from Fat 150

% Daily Value*

Total Fat 17g — **26%**

Saturated Fat 2g — **10%**

Trans Fat 0g

Cholesterol 0mg — **0%**

Sodium 370mg — **15%**

Total Carbohydrate 38g — **13%**

Dietary Fiber 10g — **40%**

Sugars 11g

Protein 10g

Asian-Style Flavored Rice

By: Alyssa Moreau

6 servings

Shiitake mushrooms, dried, soaked and sliced thin	2 each
Brown rice, medium- or short-grain, rinsed	1 1/2 cups
Water	3 cups
Salt	1 pinch
Kombu (dried seaweed), 7-inch piece	1 inch
Soy sauce, low-sodium	1 tbsp.
Mirin (Eden brand)	1 tbsp.
Carrot, julienned	1/4 cup
Gobo root (burdock), sliced thin on diagonal	1/4 cup
Soy chicken or marinated tofu, sliced	1/4 cup
Nori (dried seaweed), shredded	2 tbsp.
Green onions, sliced thin	1 tbsp.
Sesame seeds, toasted	1 tbsp.

1. Place first 10 ingredients in a rice cooker.
2. When done, place in serving bowl and garnish with the nori, green onions and sesame seeds.
3. Serve with blanched Asian greens, such as choy sum or bok choy, on the side.

Tip: The taproot of the young burdock plant is a common Japanese ingredient. It is best cooked as soon as it is sliced or cut before it quickly turns brown.

Nutrition Facts

Serving Size (204g)

Amount Per Serving

Calories 230   Calories from Fat 25

	% Daily Value*
Total Fat 2.5g	4%
Saturated Fat 0g	0%
Trans Fat 0g	
Cholesterol 0mg	0%
Sodium 410mg	17%
Total Carbohydrate 43g	14%
Dietary Fiber 3g	12%
Sugars 2g	
Protein 9g	

Barley-Rice "Risotto" with Kabocha and Azuki Beans

By: Alyssa Moreau

4 servings

Brown rice, short-grain, rinsed	1/3 cup
Pearl barley, rinsed	1/3 cup
Water	3 cups
Kabocha pumpkin, cut into 1-inch cubes	2 cups
Ginger, crystallized, chopped fine	1 tbsp.
Salt	3/4 tsp.
Sesame oil	1 tbsp.
Ginger, fresh, minced	2 tbsp.
Mirin (Eden brand)	2 tbsp.
Umeboshi vinegar	1 tsp.
Azuki beans, cooked, rinsed and drained (also available canned)	1 cup
Green onions, sliced on the diagonal	1/4 cup
Black sesame seeds	1 tsp.

1. Bring the water to a boil.
2. Add in the rice, barley, kabocha, crystallized ginger and salt.
3. Bring back to a boil, then reduce heat and simmer, uncovered, about 40 minutes, or until water is absorbed.
4. In a separate skillet, heat the sesame oil over medium heat and sauté the ginger for a few minutes.
5. Add in the mirin, vinegar and beans.
6. Heat through to meld the flavors then stir into the barley-rice-kabocha pot.
7. Adjust seasonings to taste.
8. Serve garnished with the green onions and sesame seeds.

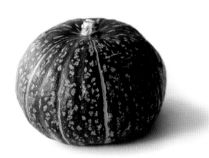

Nutrition Facts

Serving Size (166g)

Amount Per Serving

Calories 360	Calories from Fat 45

% Daily Value*

Total Fat 5g	8%
Saturated Fat 0.5g	3%
Trans Fat 0g	
Cholesterol 0mg	0%
Sodium 450mg	19%
Total Carbohydrate 66g	22%
Dietary Fiber 7g	28%
Sugars 6g	
Protein 15g	

4 servings

Water	4 1/2 cups
Dashi konbu (dried seaweed), 6-inch x 7-inch, cut in half	1 piece
Ginger, 2-inch x 1-inch, sliced and crushed slightly	1 piece
Shiitake mushrooms, dried	2 each
Lemon zest	1/4 tsp.
Bonito (fish flakes), shaved (1 oz. packets)	4 packets

1. Bring water, konbu, ginger, mushrooms and lemon zest to a boil.
2. Remove from heat, add bonito flakes, cover and let steep for 45 minutes.
3. Strain soup, squeezing as much liquid out of solids as possible.
4. Discard solids, cool stock and store in refrigerator or freeze for later use.

*Makes about 4 cups of stock

Nutrition Facts

Serving Size (287g)

Amount Per Serving

Calories 30	Calories from Fat 0

	% Daily Value*
Total Fat 0g	**0%**
Saturated Fat 0g	**0%**
Trans Fat 0g	
Cholesterol 5mg	**2%**
Sodium 75mg	**3%**
Total Carbohydrate 5g	**2%**
Dietary Fiber 1g	**4%**
Sugars 0g	
Protein 2g	

Maui Onion and Mushroom Gravy

By: Sharon Kobayashi

16 servings (2 cups)

Vegetable oil	1 tsp.
Sweet Maui onion, small dice	1 cup
Mushroom, sliced	8 oz.
Butter, unsalted	1 tbsp.
Flour	2 tbsp.
Brandy or sherry	2 tbsp.
Broth, beef, reduced-sodium	2 cups
Salt	1/2 tsp.
Sage, fresh	4 leaves
Thyme, fresh	1 to 2 sprigs
Black pepper, fresh ground	to taste

1. Cook onions in vegetable oil on medium heat until golden brown, approximately 10 minutes.
2. Add mushrooms and continue cooking.
3. When onions are deep brown and mushrooms are light brown, stir in butter.
4. When butter is melted, add flour, stirring well to coat.
5. Add brandy while stirring.
6. Add broth and salt. Bring to a boil, stirring. Reduce to a simmer.
7. Add sage and thyme, simmer for 10 minutes.
8. Remove from heat. Add a generous grinding of pepper.
9. Remove herbs before serving.

Nutrition Facts

Serving Size (63g)

Amount Per Serving

Calories 25   Calories from Fat 10

	% Daily Value*
Total Fat 1.5g	2%
Saturated Fat 0.5g	3%
Trans Fat 0g	
Cholesterol 0mg	0%
Sodium 85mg	4%
Total Carbohydrate 3g	1%
Dietary Fiber 0g	0%
Sugars 1g	
Protein 1g	

Creamy Asian Salad Dressing

By: Alyssa Moreau

8 servings

Ginger, minced	2" piece
Cilantro, chopped	1/2 cup
Garlic, minced	1 clove
Honey	2 tbsp.
White miso	1 tsp.
Cucumber, peeled and seeded, chopped in large chunks	1 each
Silken tofu (Mori-nu brand firm)	1/4 cup
Light oil	2 tbsp.
Toasted sesame oil	1 tsp.
Rice vinegar	1/4 cup
Mirin	2 tbsp.
Light soy sauce or Bragg's Liquid Aminos	1 tbsp.
Water	2 tbsp.

1. Blend all together in a blender until smooth.
2. Add water as needed to give consistency as desired.
3. Adjust seasonings to taste.

Nutrition Facts
Serving Size (83g)

Amount Per Serving

Calories 80   Calories from Fat 40

% Daily Value*

Total Fat 4.5g	7%
Saturated Fat 0g	0%
Trans Fat 0g	
Cholesterol 0mg	0%
Sodium 90mg	4%
Total Carbohydrate 9g	3%
Dietary Fiber 1g	4%
Sugars 6g	
Protein 1g	

Mango Chutney

By: Alyssa Moreau

8 to 12 servings

Mango, ripe local, peeled and cubed	2 cups
Rice vinegar	1 tbsp.
Raisins	2 tbsp.
Honey	1 tbsp.
Ginger, fresh, minced	2 tsp.
Garlic, minced	1 tsp.
Cayenne pepper	dash
Chinese parsley, minced	1 tbsp.
Cinnamon, allspice or garam masala	1/2 tsp.

1. Combine all ingredients in a small pot and bring to a boil.
2. Reduce heat and simmer for 5 to 10 minutes.
3. Break up mixture with a potato masher or fork.
4. Cool. Adjust seasonings to taste.

Nutrition Facts
Serving Size (34g)

Amount Per Serving

Calories 30   Calories from Fat 0

% Daily Value*

Total Fat 0g	0%
Saturated Fat 0g	0%
Trans Fat 0g	
Cholesterol 0mg	0%
Sodium 0mg	0%
Total Carbohydrate 8g	3%
Dietary Fiber 1g	4%
Sugars 7g	
Protein 0g	

Basic Asian Vinaigrette

By: Sharon Kobayashi

4 servings

Shallots, fresh, chopped	1 tbsp.
Balsamic vinegar	1/4 cup
Ginger, fresh, minced	1/2 tsp.
Sesame oil, toasted	1 tsp.
Soy sauce, low-sodium	1 tbsp.
Black pepper, ground	1/2 tsp. (or to taste)

1. Combine all ingredients. Stir well before using.

Nutrition Facts

Serving Size (19g)

Amount Per Serving

Calories 20   Calories from Fat 10

% Daily Value*

Total Fat 1g	**2%**
Saturated Fat 0g	**0%**
Trans Fat 0g	
Cholesterol 0mg	**0%**
Sodium 110mg	**5%**
Total Carbohydrate 2g	**1%**
Dietary Fiber 0g	**0%**
Sugars 2g	
Protein 0g	

Balsamic Dressing

By: Alyssa Moreau

4 servings

Olive oil	3 tbsp.
White balsamic vinegar	3 tbsp.
Soy sauce, low-sodium	1 tbsp.
Hawaiian Lehua or macadamia nut honey	1 tbsp.
Lime juice	1/2 lime

Nutrition Facts

Serving Size (35g)

Amount Per Serving

Calories 120   Calories from Fat 90

% Daily Value*

Total Fat 11g	**17%**
Saturated Fat 1.5g	**8%**
Trans Fat 0g	
Cholesterol 0mg	**0%**
Sodium 135mg	**6%**
Total Carbohydrate 6g	**2%**
Dietary Fiber 0g	**0%**
Sugars 6g	
Protein 0g	

Creamy Phyllo Fruit Tower

By: Alyssa Moreau

4 servings

Phyllo:

Phyllo dough, Athens brand	4 sheets
Margarine	2 tbsp.
Raw cane sugar	1 tbsp.

1. Cut phyllo sheets into strips and then rectangles or squares 3" to 4" in length. Stack 3 high, brushing lightly with melted margarine and a bit of sugar between layers. (Allow 3 of these stacks per person; for 4 people use 12 stacks of 3 layers.) Place on non-stick or parchment layered baking sheet and bake at 350 degrees for about 10 minutes or until lightly browned and crisp. Allow to cool, then store in an airtight container for up to 3 days.

Cream:

Cottage cheese, non-fat	1 1/2 cups
Cream cheese, low-fat	1/2 cup
Yogurt, low-fat, plain or vanilla	1 cup
Lemon zest	1 tsp.
Lemon juice	2 tbsp.
Vanilla	1 tsp.
Lemon flavor (optional)	1 tsp.
Honey or agave nectar	3 tbsp.
Guar gum (optional)*	1/8 tsp.
Fresh fruit of choice, 1/2" dice	2 cups

1. Combine all of the cream ingredients in a blender or food processor and blend until smooth. Adjust flavors to taste. If desired, organic margarine and raw cane sugar (turbinado) can be used for this recipe.
2. Cut up fruit and set aside in bowl.
3. When ready to serve, place 1 layer of phyllo on serving plate and top with spoonful of creamy filling. Top with fruit. Add another phyllo layer, creamy filling and fruit. Repeat one more time. Serve immediately.

Fresh Fruit Suggestion: Mango, papaya, honeydew, cantaloupe, strawberry, kiwi fruit

* Guar gum is a thickener. It helps to bind and emulsify. Available at local health food stores.

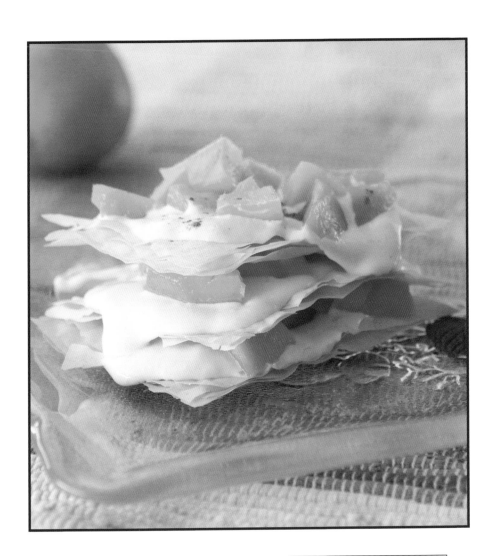

Nutrition Facts

Serving Size (202g)

Amount Per Serving

Calories 250   Calories from Fat 70

% Daily Value*

Total Fat 8g	**12**%
Saturated Fat 3g	**15**%
Trans Fat 0.5g	
Cholesterol 15mg	**5**%
Sodium 390mg	**16**%
Total Carbohydrate 33g	**11**%
Dietary Fiber 1g	**4**%
Sugars 24g	
Protein 12g	

Orange Panacotta with Fresh Papaya · By: Sharon Kobayashi

4 servings

Milk, low-fat	1 cup
Gelatin	1 1/2 tsp.
Cream cheese, reduced-fat	1 oz.
Honey	2 tbsp.
Orange juice concentrate	2 tbsp.
Vanilla	1 tsp.
Papayas, large, halved and seeded	2 each

Serving suggestion: Serve topped with orange slices and/or other seasonal fruit.

1. Soak gelatin in 1/4 cup milk for 5 minutes. (Soaking gelatin in liquid is also called "blooming.")
2. Bring remaining milk to a boil.
3. Add dissolved gelatin to boiling milk, stirring.
4. Turn off heat, stir in cream cheese until melted.
5. Pour mixture into a mixing bowl.
6. Whisk in honey, orange juice and vanilla.
7. Pour 1/4 cup into each papaya half. Refrigerate until set, about 2 hours.
8. Cover with plastic wrap and let rest overnight.

Tip: Before filling, make sure papaya halves sit level, slicing the bottom to create a flat surface if necessary. Size of papayas varies. If using a large papaya, slice off excess fruit after panacotta is set. If fruit is small, scoop out a little of the fruit—scooping the sides to create a lip at the top helps to contain the panacotta.

Nutrition Facts

Serving Size (278g)

Amount Per Serving

Calories 170	Calories from Fat 25

	% Daily Value*
Total Fat 2.5g	4%
Saturated Fat 1.5g	8%
Trans Fat 0g	
Cholesterol 10mg	3%
Sodium 75mg	3%
Total Carbohydrate 34g	11%
Dietary Fiber 3g	12%
Sugars 25g	
Protein 5g	

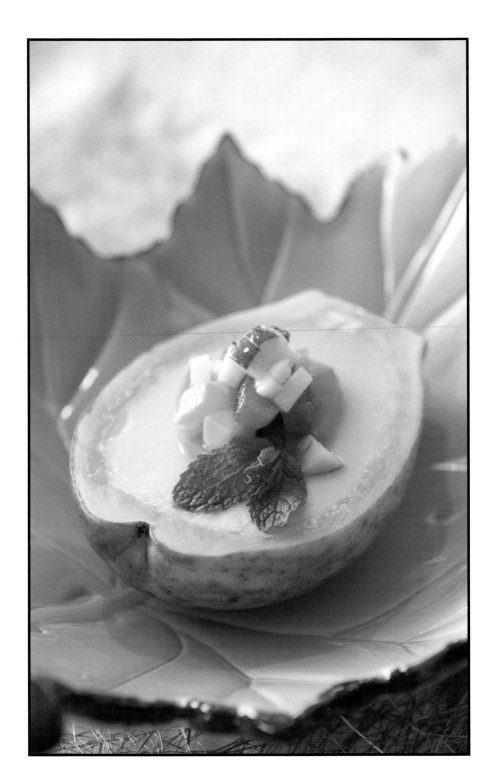

6 to 8 servings

Whole-wheat pastry flour	1 1/2 cups	Baking soda	1/2 tsp.
Dry egg replacer (Ener-G or BiPro)	2 tbsp.	Light oil	1/4 cup
Cinnamon	1/2 tsp.	Apple juice (as needed)	1/4 to 1/2 cup
Allspice or nutmeg	1/4 tsp.	Agave nectar or honey	1/3 cup
Clove	1/4 tsp.	Vanilla	1 tsp.
Salt	1/4 tsp.	Mango, diced	1 cup
Baking powder	1 tsp.		

1. Combine the dry ingredients in a large mixing bowl.
2. Separately, combine the liquid ingredients, except mango, then mix into the dry.
3. Add in the mango. Stir all until just combined. (You want the consistency to be like a thin pancake batter.)
4. Pour into an oiled 8"x8" or 9" pie plate. Bake at 350 degrees for 20 to 25 minutes. (Adding in a small pan of water to the oven helps the cake to maintain its moisture.)
5. Cool.

Frosting:

Liliko'i (passion fruit) juice, fresh (if possible) or frozen concentrate	3 to 4 tbsp.
Cream cheese, low-fat	1/2 cup
Mori-Nu extra firm silken tofu	1/2 cup
Vanilla	1 tsp.
Agave nectar or honey	2 to 3 tbsp.
Salt	1/8 tsp.

1. Combine all ingredients in a food processor or blender and process until smooth.
2. Taste and adjust flavors as desired.
3. Spread over cool cake.
4. Top with chopped macadamia nuts or more mango, if desired.

Nutrition Facts	
Serving Size (164g)	
Amount Per Serving	
Calories 360	Calories from Fat 130
	% Daily Value*
Total Fat 14g	22%
Saturated Fat 3g	15%
Trans Fat 0g	
Cholesterol 10mg	3%
Sodium 420mg	18%
Total Carbohydrate 52g	17%
Dietary Fiber 3g	12%
Sugars 29g	
Protein 8g	

Okinawan Sweet Potato-Haupia (Coconut Frosting) Pie

By: Alyssa Moreau

6 to 8 servings

Crust:

Whole-wheat pastry flour	1 cup	Light oil	3 tbsp.
Baking powder	1/2 tsp.	Agave nectar or honey	1 tbsp.
Cinnamon	1/2 tsp.	Water	2 to 3 tbsp.
Salt	1/8 tsp.		

1. Combine dry ingredients in a mixing bowl. Mix well.
2. Separately, stir together the wet ingredients then pour over the dry mixture. Combine to form a ball.
3. Place on a flour-coated board and roll out into a circle.
4. Place in 9" pie plate. Bake at 350 degrees for 10 minutes. Cool on rack.

Filling:

Okinawan sweet potato, cooked, mashed	2 cups	Agave nectar or honey	3 tbsp.
		Vanilla	1 tsp.
Milk, low-fat, or soy or rice milk	1/2 cup	Salt	1/8 tsp.

1. Combine all ingredients in a food processor and blend just until lumps have disappeared.
2. If too thick, add some water until it blends well.
3. Fill crust and smooth top. Bake at 350 degrees for 30 minutes. Cool on rack.

Haupia Topping:

Coconut milk	1/2 cup
Water	1/2 cup
Cornstarch or arrowroot	1 1/2 tbsp.
Agave nectar	2 to 4 tbsp.
Salt	1/8 tsp.
Ginger, mashed	1/2" piece

1. Combine the haupia topping mixture in a medium pot and whisk over medium-high heat until thickened.
2. Pour over semi-cool filling of pie and refrigerate until chilled and firm.

Tip: Good made the day ahead to let flavors meld and allow the haupia to gel.

Nutrition Facts

Serving Size (231g)

Amount Per Serving

Calories 340   Calories from Fat 100

	% Daily Value*
Total Fat 12g	18%
Saturated Fat 4g	20%
Trans Fat 0g	
Cholesterol 0mg	0%
Sodium 240mg	10%
Total Carbohydrate 57g	19%
Dietary Fiber 6g	24%
Sugars 26g	
Protein 5g	

Chilled Lychee and Almond Soup
By: Sharon Kobayashi

4 servings

White wine, Gewürztraminer preferred	1 cup
Pears, peeled, seeded, diced	2 each
Almond milk, vanilla-flavored	3 cups
Cornstarch	2 tsp.
Lychee, peeled, pitted and halved	1 lb.
Sugar	2 tbsp.
Sour cream, light	1/2 cup
Mint leaves, minced or cut into thin strips	8 each

1. Poach pears in wine until tender (about 10 minutes), cool and blend until smooth.
2. Return pears to the pot, add almond milk, reserving 2 tbsp.
3. Bring mix to a boil, mix reserved milk with cornstarch.
4. Stir in cornstarch slurry, boil for a minute.
5. Reduce to a simmer and cook another 10 minutes.
6. Add lychee and sugar and simmer another 5 minutes.
7. Remove from heat and cool completely. Refrigerate overnight.
8. Divide into 4 portions, top each with 2 tbsp. of sour cream and mint.

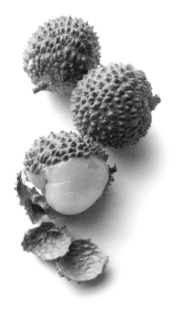

Nutrition Facts
Serving Size (475g)

Amount Per Serving

Calories 300　　　Calories from Fat 50

	% Daily Value*
Total Fat 5g	**8%**
Saturated Fat 2g	**10%**
Trans Fat 0.5g	
Cholesterol 10mg	**3%**
Sodium 140mg	**6%**
Total Carbohydrate 52g	**17%**
Dietary Fiber 5g	**20%**
Sugars 43g	
Protein 4g	

Tropical Granita
By: Sharon Kobayashi

6 servings

Pineapple, diced 1-inch	4 cups
Apple banana, diced 1-inch	1 each
Dark rum	1/4 cup
Sugar	1/4 cup
Evaporated skim milk	1 cup
Cardamom, ground	1/4 tsp.

1. Blend all ingredients, pour into a shallow pan.
2. Place in the freezer until almost frozen.
3. Remove from freezer, break into flakes with a fork.
4. Store in a covered container in freezer until ready to serve.

Nutrition Facts

Serving Size (202g)

Amount Per Serving

Calories 140   Calories from Fat 5

	% Daily Value*
Total Fat 0g	0%
Saturated Fat 0g	0%
Trans Fat 0g	
Cholesterol 0mg	0%
Sodium 55mg	2%
Total Carbohydrate 35g	12%
Dietary Fiber 1g	4%
Sugars 26g	
Protein 4g	

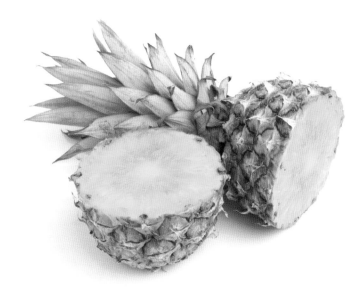

The authors and editors of this book do not endorse, nor intend to promote, any particular products. Certain brand names are mentioned in the recipes due to their products' acceptable level of nutrients such as sodium, cholesterol, saturated fat, etc. that are the focus of the DASH eating plan. Other product brands are mentioned as they are found by the chef authors to impart certain desirable quality in terms of taste, appearance and consistency to the dishes in the course of recipe development. 🍅

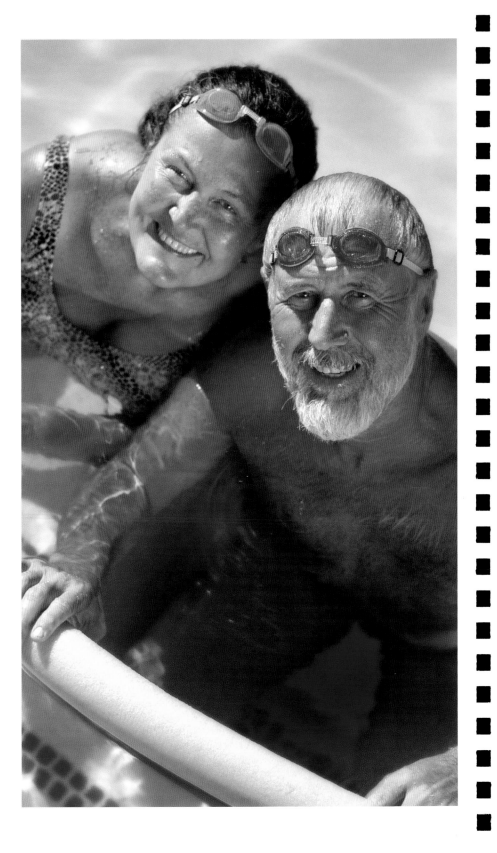

Chapter 6

The DASHing Kupuna
The DASH Eating Plan and Active Aging

Compiled by
Cullen Hayashida, Ph.D.
Aging and Long-Term Care Training Initiative Coordinator
Kapiʻolani Community College

and

Daniel Leung, A.S. (Culinary Arts), M.S.W.
Education Specialist
Kapiʻolani Community College

W e all wish to age gracefully. Who would not want to continue to be active and spend time with their children, their grandchildren or their friends? Who would not want to engage in favorite pastime activities, in get-togethers for family meals or other seasonal festivities in their retirement years? Nutritious food and physical exercise are two important factors that will determine whether you can achieve that state of well-being that we call active aging.

Active Aging

According to the World Health Organization, Active Aging is "the process of optimizing opportunities for health, participation and security in order to enhance quality of life as people age." Following retirement, we all wish to remain independent with physical activities, lifelong learning and social participation. Active aging requires taking personal responsibility for our physical and mental health in order to prevent long-term care and premature institutional placement.

Here are seven facets of successful Active Aging:

1. **Nutritional Fitness** – "You are what you eat." Pay special attention to your nutritional well-being with tips from this book. Drink water, reduce fat, eat more fiber, reduce salt intake and don't forget your vitamins!
2. **Physical Fitness** – "Use it or lose it!" Regular exercise maintains fitness, stimulates the mind, improves your regularity and generally enhances the quality of your life.
3. **Medical Fitness** – "No one knows yourself like you do." Watch your weight. Don't smoke, do control your cholesterol and blood pressure. Take your meds. Inform your doctor of changes.
4. **Mental Fitness** – "If you think that you are old, you are old." The great enemies to a healthy senior mind are depression, loneliness and boredom. Social activities, hobbies and exercise are great anti-depressants. Stay active and volunteer your time.
5. **Financial Fitness** – "Assure that your retirement years are golden years." Anticipate about 30 years of life without employment. Plan for how pen-

sion, social security, home equity, deferred compensation, insurance, reverse mortgage and other strategies will keep you financially fit.

6. **Consumer/Legal Fitness** – "Beware of scams." Seniors are often targets of high-pressure tactics and scams. Protect your records. If it's too good to be true, it probably is a scam.

7. **Spiritual Fitness** – "It is better to give than to receive." What will you do with the rest of your life? How do you wish to be remembered? Do an assessment of your life goals and challenge yourself by assisting the next generation or your community. Having purpose in life will energize you.

Nutritional Callenges for Older Adults

Good nutrition is especially important to older adults, by helping them to maintain strength, stave off disease, illness and frailty. However, individuals often experience great nutritional challenges as they age. According to Dr. Susan Calvert Finn, past president of the American Dietetic Association, older adults are often at high risk for malnutrition due to the following:

- Decreased body organ function affects the absorption, movement, metabolism and elimination of nutrients.
- Decreased physical mobility and dexterity lessen a person's ability to access, prepare and eat food.
- Poor dental conditions have caused 50 percent of Americans age 65 and older to lose their teeth, and many others have teeth in poor condition or have poorly fitting dentures. This severely limits food choices and food intake.
- Multiple prescription drug use interferes with digestion, absorption and the elimination of nutrients that lead to nutrient deficiencies.
- Social isolation, boredom, depression and loneliness can result in loss of appetite and unwillingness to prepare adequate meals, leading to malnutrition.
- Poverty or near-poverty conditions force millions of elderly persons to choose between housing expenses and enough food, and/or prescription drugs and proper nutrition.
- Diminished senses (sight, smell and taste) affect nutritional intake and nutritional health.

According to Finn's research, up to 50 percent of all older adults living independently within a community have some type of nutritional deficiency. Far too often, signs of malnutrition and dehydration are mistaken as signs of aging, since someone who is malnourished or dehydrated will appear lethargic, confused and/or disoriented. Also older adults often have chronic health problems, such as hypertension, diabetes, osteoporosis, heart disease and cancer that can be exacerbated by poor nutrition.

Yet, proper nutrition has been found to be successful in the prevention and treatment of these conditions (U.S. House of Representatives Select Committee on Aging 1992b). A useful tool to screen the nutritional health of older adults is the publication *Screening Older Americans' Nutritional Health: Current Practices and Future Possibilities*. This publication is available for $5. See sidebar for details.

> **Nutritional Screening Initiative**
> 2626 Pennsylvania Ave., NW, Suite 301
> Washington D.C. 20037
>
> **Also, a fact sheet entitled** *Determine Your Nutritional Health* **is available, free of charge, by calling the Area Agency on Aging of West Michigan. They can be reached at (616) 456-5664.**

What Is Good Nutrition for an Older Adult?

Older adults generally have the same nutritional requirements as young people. The Recommended Daily Allowance (RDA) nutritional guidelines for adults are divided into only two categories, those 25 to 50 years old, and 51 years old and older. However, because seniors are less active, their caloric intake needs to decrease with age. Therefore, it is imperative that their food be denser in nutritional value. As of 1989, the RDA for a 50- to 60-year-old is 1,700 calories per day where the RDA for a 70- to 80-year-old is only 1,500 calories per day, and somewhere in between for a 60- to 70-year-old.

According to the U.S. Department of Agriculture, and U.S. Department of Health and Human Services publication, *Nutrition and Your Health: Dietary Guidelines for Americans* (Fifth Edition, 2000), Americans should:

Aim for Fitness ...
- Aim for a healthy weight.
- Be physically active each day.

Build a Healthy Base ...
- Use the DASH eating plan and the Food Pyramid to guide your food choices.
- Choose a variety of grains daily, especially whole grains.
- Choose a variety of fruits and vegetables daily.
- Stock your refrigerator and pantry with food appropriate to your health status.

Choose Sensibly ...
- Choose a diet that is low in saturated fat and cholesterol and moderate in total fat.
- Choose beverages and foods with less sugar.
- Choose and prepare foods with less salt.
- If you drink alcoholic beverages, do so in moderation.

A free copy of the publication *Nutrition and Your Health: Dietary Guidelines for Americans* can be obtained from the USDA via the internet at www.usda.gov/cnpp or you can request a copy for 50 cents by writing to:

Federal Citizen Information Center U.S. General Services Administration
1800 F Street NW, Room G142
Washington, DC 20405
202-501-1794
www.pueblo.gsa.gov/

Due to chronic conditions such as osteoporosis, and the prevalence of anemia among the elderly, the diet of an older adult should also include an adequate amount of calcium and iron.

Sharing a Meal: The Value of Mealtime

You can use the recipes in this book for the entire family, from older adults who are concerned about their nutritional intake to younger family members who want to eat healthy and be fit. So for those who are caring for their parents with special dietary restrictions, you will not need to cook separately for yourself and your older parents. For those older adults who live on their own, these recipes are also easy to use for single or double servings.

Older adults have traditionally viewed mealtime as a time of family togetherness. Mealtime was a time of socialization and bonding. This is why many isolated older adults who live alone have decreased appetites and no longer eat a nutritionally balanced diet. Seniors who eat out of loneliness, depression and boredom also tend to eat food that is less nutritious and therefore adds to a weight problem, which in turn raises their risk of falling if they become obese.

Therefore, finding the time to eat with others is a very important part of the nutritional health of older adults.

Think of the pleasure derived from preparing and serving a healthy and tasty meal to others who gratefully enjoy it. For those who are living on their own, invite family, friends or a neighbor to eat with you.

Mealtime Planning Tips

As stated earlier, eating alone and cooking for only one or two can be a difficult experience for many older adults. Perhaps the following mealtime planning tips from dietician Paula Kerr can be helpful:

Before grocery shopping:
- Check your supply of staple foods, like bread products, meats and canned foods.
- Cut coupons from magazines and newspapers.
- Make a list of food you need to buy.
- Eat a meal or snack before you go shopping.

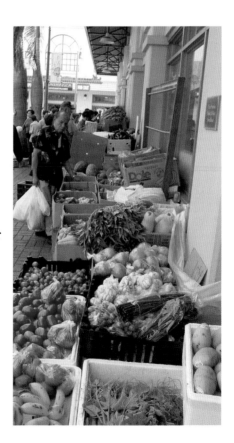

At the store:
- Look at the store advertisement for food that is on sale.
- Choose low-cost protein foods, such as fish, eggs, milk, chicken and legumes (dry beans).
- Choose generic brand food.
- Decide which size package is right for you—remember, bigger packages are not always the best value.

- Do not buy many ready-to-eat products; they are more expensive.
- Share large packages with a friend.
- Check all packages for freshness and expiration dates.
- Look for local, farm-fresh products at farmers markets or Chinatown markets. Be wary of the value associated with imported "natural, healthy or organic" foods that can be a lot more expensive.
- Buy fresh produce only in the amounts you need.
- Consider asking the butcher to cut smaller pieces of meat for you.

In preparing foods:
- Make large amounts of foods that you like at one time.
- Refrigerate some of it to eat the next day.
- Freeze some of the food by putting it in small containers.
- Write the date and type of food on it before freezing.

At mealtimes:
- Eat regular meals and snacks each day.
- Eat with a friend or family member often.
- Listen to relaxing music while eating.
- Enjoy the food you are eating.
- Eat slowly to help with digestion.
- Refrigerate or throw away any leftovers right after you are finished eating.

Source: Kent County Resource Roadmap on Successful Aging, *Grand Rapids, Michigan*
http://web.grcc.cc.mi.us/olc/Resource%20Roadmap%20(PDF).pdf

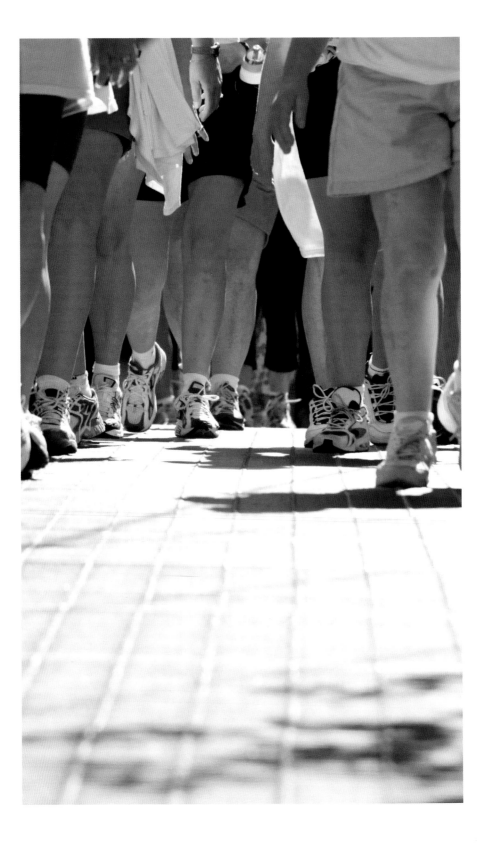

Chapter 7

A DASH to Action

Douglas Crowell, M.S., C.S.C.S., C-PT
Coordinator for Exercise and Sport Science
Kapiʻolani Community College

Master's degree in *Adult Fitness and Cardiac Rehabilitation*
and a Bachelor's degree in *Physical Education-Exercise Specialist*

Certified Personal Trainer
National Academy of Sports Medicine
and the *American Council on Exercise*

Certified Strength and Conditioning Specialist
National Strength and Conditioning Association

Consider this statement:

Do 30 minutes of moderate-intensity activity every day.

The American College of Sports Medicine (ACSM), the Center for Disease Control (CDC) and the Surgeon General have been proposing this for years.

Why? Research has shown that this amount of activity can improve many aspects of our health, including blood pressure.

How much and how often?

Based upon extensive research related to exercise and hypertension, the American College of Sports Medicine in 2004 proposed the following exercise prescription for those with hypertension:

TABLE 1

Frequency of activity:	on most, preferably all, days of the week
Intensity of activity:	moderate intensity
Time of activity:	≥ 30 minutes of continuous or accumulated physical activity per day
Type of activity:	primarily endurance physical activity supplemented by resistance exercise

American College of Sports Medicine (2004). Position Stand on Exercise and Hypertension. *Medicine and Science in Sports and Exercise,* 36, 533-553.

So, take a look at the amount of exercise that you need to improve your blood pressure.

Always check with your doctor prior to beginning an exercise program. Once you get permission from your doctor, consider the following activities that are considered moderate intensity (Table 2). However, for some people, these moderate activities may be too intense. They aren't right for everyone.

Persons with physical disabilities should consult with their physician, physical therapist, exercise physiologist or certified personal trainer to help them decide which exercises are best.

Do what you enjoy!!

Here is a list of moderate-intensity activities to consider.

TABLE 2

Walking at a moderate or brisk pace of 2.5 to 4.5 mph on a level surface inside or outside such as:	Dancing	Coaching football, soccer, basketball
	Water aerobics	Slow ballroom dancing
	Slimnastics	Hula
	Light calisthenics at home	Surfing
Walking at the mall	Snorkeling	Body surfing
Walking to work	Light rowing or paddling	Body board surfing
Walking to the store	Boxing—punching bag	Softball
Walking the dog	Table tennis	Skateboarding
Walking during a work break	Tennis—doubles	Playing kids' games with children
Walking on a treadmill	Golf—carrying clubs	Bowling
Walking downstairs or down a hill	Horseback riding	Raking lawn
Hiking	Archery	Gardening and planting trees
In-line skating, leisurely	Badminton	Water volleyball
Bicycling 5 to 10 mph	Hatha yoga	Leisurely swimming
Stationary cycling at moderate effort	Tai chi	Playing frisbee
	Juggling	Sailing
Aerobics, low-impact	Horseshoe pitching	Hunting
	Shooting baskets	

Table adapted from Ainsworth et al. *Compendium of physical activities: classification of energy costs of human physical activities.* Medicine and Science in Sports and Exercise, *1193, 25 (1): 71-80 and from* Physical Activity for Everyone: Recommendations at www.cdc.gov/nccdphp/dnpa/physical/recommendations/index.htm

Although research has shown that higher-intensity activities and longer durations offer more health benefits, these activities are a great starting point. Another important question to ask yourself is how you feel while doing these activities. Choose activities with minimum risk that are easy to do. Also, choose activities that are always available regardless of weather, e.g., indoor cycling, mall walking.

To see if the intensity is moderate for you, use Table 3. This chart will help you rate the intensity of the activity that you choose to do for 30 minutes. If you rate the intensity of the activity between three and five, it is of moderate intensity. If you rate the activity 6 or above, slow down until your body becomes more conditioned to handle it.

If you can't carry on a conversation or you are gasping for air, slow down so that you can talk while you are doing the activity. It is very important to listen to your body while you are exercising. Remember, exercise doesn't have to be hard to be beneficial to your health and to help you lower your blood pressure.

Do What's Right For You

This table allows you to gauge the intensity of the exercise that you plan to do for your regular physical activity routine. Rate how challenging the exercise feels to you on a scale ranging from 0 to 10. If your answer to the question "Are you able to:" is a "no," then the intensity of the exercise would be at a higher level on the scale. For example: If you can not talk while you are doing the exercise, then it would be a 6 on the scale and is close to being a very heavy routine.

TABLE 3

Intensity:		Are you able to:	Is your breathing:
0	Nothing at all		
0.5	Extremely weak		
1	Very weak		
2	Weak (light)	Whistle/sing	Light
3	Moderate		
4	Somewhat strong		
5	Strong (heavy)	Talk	Heavier, but you can talk
6			
7	Very strong		
8			
9		Breathe in without gasping	Real heavy and you can't talk
10	Extremely strong		

Adapted from: Borg, G. (1982). Psychological Bases of Perceived Exertion. *Medicine and Science in Sports and Exercise, 14,* 377-387.

Some physicians may ask you to monitor your heart rate during exercise. This is another way of measuring the intensity of an activity. Please check with your physician for an appropriate heart rate for your exercise intensity.

Remember to take three to five minutes before activity to warm up your body and exercising muscles, e.g., light calisthenics. This will prepare your body for your activity. Or start at an easy pace and gradually increase the intensity slowly. And don't forget to cool down for three to five minutes following your activity. It is a good way to let your body slowly wind down from any activity. The cool down is a good time to include some stretching exercises.

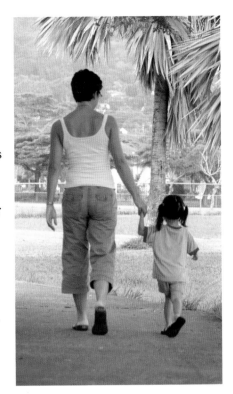

Q & A: Workout Basics

Question: How many times per week (frequency) should I move my body?
Answer: At least five days, preferably every day of the week.

Question: How hard (intensity) should the activity be?
Answer: Moderate intensity.

Question: How long (time) should I do the activity?
Answer: Do your activity of choice for at least 30 minutes. OR you can even break it up into smaller bouts throughout the day. For example, walk for 10 minutes, 3 times a day. Although 30 minutes or more of continuous exercise is recommended, especially for weight loss, breaking up your exercise is a nice option to consider.

Question: What kind (type) of activity should I do?
Answer: If you noticed from the list of moderate activities, most of the activities typically involve using many muscles at the same time. In other words, any activities that use large muscle groups continuously are the best choice.

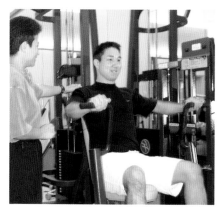

However, research has shown that in addition to these types of endurance exercises, resistance training (strength training) may be helpful in lowering blood pressure.

The American College of Sports Medicine has suggested that the following **guidelines for resistance training** is appropriate for people with hypertension:

1. Do resistance training two to three non-consecutive days per week.
2. Do one set of each exercise per workout.
3. Do 10 to 20 repetitions per set of each exercise, but do not strain or perform at maximum level.
4. Do eight to 10 separate exercises that train the major muscles of the hips, thighs, legs, chest, shoulders, arms, back and abdomen.
5. Use free weights, machines and bands as forms of resistance training.

The American College of Sports Medicine also recommends:
A. Use good form when doing the exercises.
B. Do not hold your breath because that can cause excessive increases in blood pressure.

You should also limit your overhead movements and avoid excessive gripping of equipment. It might be a good idea to check with a certified physical therapist or fitness professional who has some experience working with people with hypertension. And always check with your physician prior to beginning any resistance training program.

Flexibility exercises, such as stretching, can also be incorporated into your activity plan. Stretching and flexibility exercises improve the range of motion of a joint and enhance muscular performance. Improving your range of motion in your joints may decrease your risk of injury. Stretching exercises can improve your posture. Stretching exercises can also can help reduce muscular tension, which promotes relaxation. The best time to stretch is when your muscles are warm. So, it's best to stretch following your exercise or physical activity.

The American College of
Sports Medicine also rec-
ommends that you should
stretch the major muscle
groups two to three days
per week. Static stretches
be held for 10 to 30 seconds
and repeated four times
per muscle group. Again, it
might be a good idea to check
with a physical therapist or
certified fitness professional
before attempting any of the
exercises.

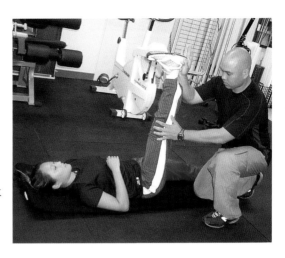

Here's how you start ...
So are you ready to exercise and get more activity in your life?

Beginning to exercise is a major lifestyle change for many people. It involves
learning new behaviors in order to support that lifestyle change. Research
suggests that people actually go through stages when they decide to make
changes in their life.

TABLE 4

Most people go through a 5-stage process with regards to making any behavior changes in their life. These stages can be simply described as:	
STAGE 1	No interest in changing behavior
STAGE 2	Thinking about changing a behavior but haven't committed to it
STAGE 3	Preparing to change a behavior by making a plan of action
STAGE 4	Taking action and practicing behaviors to maintain the plan
STAGE 5	Maintaining the plan and having it feel automatic (a habit)

Adapted from: Prochaska, J.O. et al. (1994). *Changing for Good*. New York: William
Morrow.

This will definitely get you going.

The following suggestions may be helpful in changing your exercise behavior:

- Make a list of any reasons why you don't exercise and think of ways to overcome them.
- Reflect about how you might get sick if you don't get any exercise.
- List the pros and cons of getting more exercise in your life.
- Visualize how your life will be better with more exercise.
- Identify convenient resources in your community.
- Discuss your plans with people who will give you positive support.

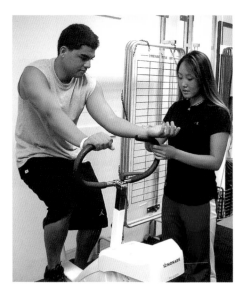

- Write a contract for yourself.
- Map out various walking routes in your neighborhood.
- Make a New Year's resolution and get support from your friends and family to stick with it.
- Post your exercise plans on the refrigerator.
- Post motivation signs and affirmations about your plans at work.
- See if a friend would like to join you in your plans to become more active.
- Keep a schedule of your available times to exercise throughout the week.
- Ask yourself, what are the benefits of getting more exercise?
- Analyze if the sacrifice of time to exercise is worth it.
- Learn more about the benefits of physical activity.
- Find an exercise support group, e.g., tai chi group, walking group.
- Ask yourself: Have I moved my body for 30 minutes today?
- Locate parks and walking trails in your area.
- Schedule exercise time in your daily plan or time slots for exercise.
- Plan ahead and write your activities on a calendar.
- Hire a certified personal trainer.
- Treat your exercise time like an appointment that you can't miss.
- Burn a CD of your favorite music to use when you are walking.
- Try to exercise when the kids are not around.
- Hire a babysitter or find facilities with child care services.

- Select activities that require minimal equipment, e.g., walking.
- Use appropriate clothing and shoes for all activities.
- Tell your family that you will walk for 20 minutes when you get home from work.
- Keep a log or diary of your activity and your progress.
- Have a back up plan in case of bad weather.
- Buy a pedometer to keep track of your steps and set a goal of 10,000 steps per day.
- Vary your activities both for so you don't get bored.
- Use countering behaviors such as walking with your spouse rather than watching TV.
- Reward yourself with gifts when you keep to your plan.
- Make bets with friends that you will maintain your exercise plan for a certain period of time.

Exercise and getting physically active is a life-long endeavor. It is always a good idea to look at all your options and be creative (Table 5). Get support from a friend, family member, colleague, or a supportive group. Support is a key part of maintaining your exercise behavior. And have fun!

If it hurts, don't do it!!
Are there any precautions to exercising or participating in exercise?

If the following symptoms occur before, during, or after exercise, contact your physician before you continue your activity plan.

1. Chest pain or other discomfort in the upper body, including the arm, neck or jaw, during exercise. The discomfort may be an aching, burning, tightness or sensation of fullness in those areas.
2. Fainting spell or feeling of faintness during or after exercise.
3. Shortness of breath that continues following five minutes of exercise.
4. Discomfort in bones and joints either during or after exercise.
5. Nausea after exercise.
6. Chronic fatigue throughout the day following exercise.
7. Sleeplessness.
8. Uncomfortable cramps and pains in the leg muscles during exercise.
9. If monitoring your blood pressure at home, a resting systolic > 200 mm Hg or resting diastolic blood pressure of > 110 mm Hg.
10. If monitoring your blood sugar, if you have a blood glucose > 300 mg per dl.
11. Any orthopedic conditions that prevents you from exercising.

American College of Sports Medicine (2006). *ACSM's Guidelines for Exercise Testing and Prescription* (7th ed.). Philadelphia: Lippincott, Williams & Wilkins.

See how easy it is ...

How do I get more spontaneous activity in my life? Consider these options:

TABLE 5

Park as far away from your destination as possible and walk.
Take a walk during your lunch break.
Take the stairs. Use the stairs whenever you can.
Get off the bus several bus stops or blocks away from destination.
Take fitness breaks at work and go for quick five minute walks.
Exercise while watching TV.
Keep a pair of walking shoes at your work or in the car.
Consider buying a piece of exercise equipment for your home—e.g., a treadmill.
Make your activities social—maybe regular Saturday morning walks with friends.
Always walk in the mall for 30 minutes first prior to shopping.
Take walks in the airport if you have time between flights.
If at the beach, go for a swim or bring a volleyball or Frisbee to play with the kids.
Get to your job 30 minutes earlier and take a walk before you start.
When traveling, stay in places that have fitness centers, pools, etc.
Contact your local Parks and Recreation Department, YMCA or community organization to find out if they offer any programs or exercise classes that may interest you. For example: www.honolulu.gov/parks/programs www.ymcahonolulu.org

Chapter 8

Hawai'i Nutrition & Seasonality Charts

Hawai'i Fruits Seasonality Chart

M - Indicates MODERATE availability • **P** - Indicates PEAK availability

	JAN	FEB	MAR	APR	MAY	JUN	JUL	AUG	SEP	OCT	NOV	DEC
Atemoya	M	M						M	M	P	P	P
Avocado	P	P	M	M					M	M	P	P
Banana	M	M	M	M	M	P	P	P	P	P	M	M
Cantaloupe					M	P	P	P	M			
Honeydew					M	P	P	P	P			
Lime	P	P	P			P	P	P	P	P	P	P
Longan	M	M	M	M	M	M	M	P	P	P	M	M
Lychee	M	M	M	M	P	P	P	P	P	M	M	M
Mango			P	P	P	P	P	P	P	P	P	
Orange	P	P	P	P	M	M	M	M	P	P	P	P
Papaya	M	M	P	P	P	P	P	P	P	P	P	M
Persimmon										P	P	M
Pineapple	M	M	M	P	P	P	P	P	P	M	M	M
Rambutan	P	P	P							P	P	P
Strawberry	P	P	P	P	M	M	M			M	M	M
Starfruit	M	M	M	M					M	M	M	M
Tangerine	P	M								M	P	P
Watermelon					M	P	P	P	P	M		

Source: Hawai'i Agriculture & Food Products Directory • www.Hawaiiag.org/hdoa/

These charts were developed by the College of Tropical Agriculture and Human Resources at the University of Hawai'i in collaboration with the Hawai'i Department of Agriculture and the Hawai'i Farm Bureau Federation.

Hawai'i Vegetables Seasonality Chart

M - Indicates MODERATE availability • **P** - Indicates PEAK availability

	JAN	FEB	MAR	APR	MAY	JUN	JUL	AUG	SEP	OCT	NOV	DEC
Beans	M	M	M	P	P	P	P	P	M	M	M	M
Bittermelon	M	P	P	P	P	P	M	M				
Burdock	M	M	M				M	P	P	P	P	P
Cabbage, Chinese	P	P	P	P	P	P	P	P	M	M	M	M
Cabbage, Head	M	P	P	P	P	P	M	M	M	M	M	M
Cabbage, Asian	M	M	M				M	P	P	P	P	P
Celery		M	M	P	P	P	P	P	M	M		
Corn, Sweet	M	P	P	P	P	P	M	M	M	M	P	P
Cucumber	M	M	M	P	P	P	P	P	M	M	M	M
Daikon	M	M	M	M	M	M	P	P	P	P	M	M
Eggplant	M	M	P	P	P	P	M	M	M	M	M	M
Ginger Root		M	M	P	P	P	P	P	M	M	M	
Heart of Palm	P	P	P	P	P	P	P	P	P	P	P	P
Herbs	M	M	M	M	M	M	M	M	M	M	M	M
Lettuce, Baby Greens	M	M	M			M	M	P	P	P	P	P
Lettuce, Romaine	M	M	M	M	M	P	P	P	P	M	M	M
Lettuce, Leaf	M	M	P	P	P	P	P	M	M	M	M	M
Lü'au (Taro) Leaf				M	M	P	P	P	P	M	M	
Mushrooms	P	P	P	P	P	P	P	P	P	P	P	P
Onion, Round			M	P	P	P	P	P	M	M		
Onion, Green	M	M	M	M	M	M	P	P	P	P	M	M
Parsley, American	M	M	P	P	P	P	M	M				
Pepper, Green	M	M	M	P	P	P	P	P	M	M	M	M
Potato, Sweet	M	P	P	P	P	P	M	M				
Pumpkin	M	M	M			M	M	P	P	P	P	P
Sprouts	P	P	P	P	P	P	P	P	P	P	P	P
Squash				M	M	P	P	P	P	M	M	
Taro	M	M	P	P	P	P	P	M	M	M	P	P
Tomato	M	M	M	M	P	P	P	P	P	M	M	M
Zucchini	M	M	M			M	M	P	P	P	P	P

Source: Hawai'i Agriculture & Food Products Directory • www.Hawaiiag.org/hdoa/

Raw Fruits	Serving Size of Edible Portion (gram weight/ounce weight)	Calories	Calories from fat	Total Fat		Sodium	
				g	(%)	mg	(%)
Apple	1 medium (154 g/5.5 oz)	80	0	0	0	0	0
Avocado	California 1/5 medium (30 g/1.1 oz)	55	45	5	8	0	0
Banana	1 medium (126 g/4.5 oz)	110	0	0	0	0	0
Cantaloupe	1/4 medium (134 g/4.8 oz)	50	0	0	0	25	1
Grapefruit	1/2 medium (154 g/5.5 oz)	60	0	0	0	0	0
Grapes	3/4 cup (126 g/4.5 oz)	90	0	0	0	0	0
Honeydew Melon	1/10 medium (134 g/4.8 oz)	50	0	0	0	35	1
Kiwifruit	2 medium (148 g/5.3 oz)	100	10	1	2	0	0
Lemon	1 medium (58 g/2.1 oz)	15	0	0	0	5	0
Lime	1 medium (67 g/2.4 oz)	20	0	0	0	0	0
Nectarine	1 medium (140 g/5.0 oz)	70	0	0	0	0	0
Orange	1 medium (154g/5.5 oz)	70	0	0	0	0	0
Peach	1 medium (98 g/3.5 oz)	40	0	0	0	0	0
Pear	1 medium (166 g/5.9 oz)	100	10	1	2	0	0
Pineapple	2 slices; 3" diameter (112 g/4.0 oz)	60	0	0	0	10	0
Plums	2 medium (132 g/4.07 oz)	80	10	1	2	0	0
Strawberries	8 medium (147 g/5.3 oz)	45	0	0	0	0	0
Sweet Cherries	21 cherries; 1 cup (140 g/5.0 oz)	90	0	0	0	0	0
Tangerine	1 medium (109 g/3.9 oz)	50	0	0	0	0	0
Watermelon	1/8 medium melon; 2 cups diced pieces (280 g/10.0 oz)	80	0	0	0	10	0

Nutritional Facts for Raw Fruits

Potassium		Total Carb		Dietary Fiber		Sugars	Protein	Vitamin A	Vitamin C	Calcium	Iron
mg	(%)	g	(%)	g	(%)	g	g	(%)	(%)	(%)	(%)
170	5	22	7	5	20	16	0	2	8	0	2
170	5	3	1	3	12	0	1	0	4	0	0
400	11	29	10	4	16	21	1	0	15	0	2
280	8	12	4	1	4	11	1	100	80	2	2
230	7	16	5	6	24	10	1	15	110	2	0
240	7	23	8	1	4	23	1	2	25	2	0
310	9	13	4	1	4	12	1	2	45	0	2
480	14	24	8	4	16	16	2	2	240	6	4
90	3	5	2	1	4	1	0	0	40	2	0
75	2	7	2	2	8	0	0	0	35	0	0
300	8	16	5	2	8	12	1	4	15	0	2
260	7	21	7	7	28	14	1	2	130	6	2
190	5	10	3	2	8	9	1	2	10	0	2
210	6	25	8	4	16	17	1	0	10	2	0
115	3	16	5	1	4	13	1	0	25	2	2
220	6	19	6	2	8	10	1	6	20	0	0
270	8	12	4	4	16	8	1	0	160	2	4
300	9	22	7	3	12	19	2	2	15	2	2
180	5	15	5	3	12	12	1	0	50	4	0
230	7	27	9	2	8	25	1	20	25	2	4

This chart was developed by the College of Tropical Agriculture and Human Resources at the University of Hawai'i in collaboration with the Hawai'i Department of Health and the Hawai'i Food Industry Association.

Nutritional Facts for Raw Vegetables

Raw Vegetables	Serving Size of Edible Portion (gram weight/ounce weight)	Calories	Calories from fat	Total Fat		Sodium	
				g	(%)	mg	(%)
Asparagus	5 spears (93 g/3.3 oz)	25	0	0	0	0	0
Bell Pepper	1 medium (48 g/5.3 oz)	30	0	0	0	0	0
Broccoli	1 medium stalk (148 g/5.3 oz)	45	0	0.5	1	55	2
Carrot	1 carrot; 7" long; 1/4" diameter (78 g/2.8 oz)	35	0	0	0	40	2
Cauliflower	1/6 medium head (99 g/3.5 oz)	25	0	0	0	30	1
Celery	2 medium stalks (110 g/3.9 oz)	20	0	0	0	100	4
Cucumber	1/3 medium (99 g/3.5 oz)	15	0	0	0	0	0
Green (Snap) Beans	3/4 cup cut (83 g/3.0 oz)	25	0	0	0	0	0
Green Cabbage	1/12 medium head (84 g/3.0 oz)	25	0	0	0	20	1
Green Onion	1/4 cup chopped (25 g/0.9 oz)	10	0	0	0	5	0
Iceberg Lettuce	1/6 medium head (89 g/3.2 oz)	15	0	0	0	10	0
Leaf Lettuce	1 1/2 cups shredded (85g/3.0 oz)	15	0	0	0	30	1
Mushroom	5 medium (84 g/3.0 oz)	20	0	0	0	0	0
Onion	1 medium (148 g/5.3 oz)	60	0	0	0	5	0
Potato	1 medium (148 g/5.3 oz)	100	0	0	0	0	0
Radish	7 radishes (85 g/3.0 oz)	15	0	0	0	25	1
Summer Squash	1/2 medium (98 g/3.5 oz)	20	0	0	0	0	0
Sweet Corn	kernals from 1 medium ear (90 g/3.2 oz)	80	10	1	2	0	0
Sweet Potato	1 medium; 5" long; 2" diameter (130 g/4.6 oz)	130	0	0	0	45	2
Tomato	1 medium (148 g/5.3 oz)	35	0	0.5	1	5	0

Potassium		Total Carb		Dietary Fiber		Sugars	Protein	Vitamin A	Vitamin C	Calcium	Iron
mg	(%)	g	(%)	g	(%)	g	g	(%)	(%)	(%)	(%)
230	7	4	1	2	8	2	2	10	15	2	2
270	8	7	2	2	8	4	1	8	190	2	2
540	15	8	3	5	20	3	5	15	220	6	6
280	8	8	3	2	8	5	1	270	10	2	0
270	8	5	2	2	8	2	2	0	100	2	2
350	10	5	2	2	8	0	1	2	15	4	2
170	5	3	1	1	4	2	1	4	10	2	2
200	6	5	2	3	12	2	1	4	10	4	2
190	5	5	2	2	8	3	1	0	70	4	2
70	2	2	1	1	4	1	0	2	8	0	0
120	3	3	1	1	4	2	1	4	6	2	2
230	7	4	1	2	8	2	1	40	6	4	0
300	9	3	1	1	4	0	3	0	2	0	2
240	7	14	5	3	12	9	2	0	20	4	2
720	21	26	9	3	12	3	4	0	45	2	6
230	7	3	1	0	0	2	1	0	30	2	0
260	7	4	1	2	8	2	1	6	30	2	2
240	7	18	6	3	12	5	3	2	10	0	2
350	10	33	11	4	16	7	2	440	30	2	2
360	10	7	2	1	4	4	1	20	40	2	2

This chart was developed by the College of Tropical Agriculture and Human Resources at the University of Hawai'i in collaboration with the Hawai'i Department of Health and the Hawai'i Food Industry Association.

Contributors

American Heart Association of Hawaiʻi, contributing editor
Founded in 1924, the American Heart Association today is the nation's oldest and largest voluntary health organization dedicated to building healthier lives free of cardiovascular diseases and stroke. These diseases, America's No. 1 and No. 3 killers, and all other cardiovascular diseases claim more than 870,000 lives a year. In fiscal year 2005–06 the association invested more than $543 million in research, professional and public education, advocacy and community service programs to help all Americans live longer, healthier lives. To learn more, call 1-800-AHA-USA1 or visit www.americanheart.org.

The National Kidney Foundation of Hawaiʻi, contributing editor
The National Kidney Foundation of Hawaiʻi (NKFH), Inc. is one of 48 affiliates of the National Kidney Foundation. NKFH is a not-for-profit, volunteer-driven health agency that is governed by a local volunteer board of directors. Since its inception 12 years ago, NKFH seeks to prevent kidney diseases, improve the well-being of individuals and families affected by these diseases and increase organ transplant availability. The mission is to provide services and research for patients with kidney disease and related disorders, publishing educational materials for the general public, advocating for high quality health care, and promoting awareness of organ and tissue donation.

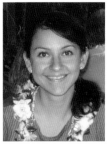

Adriana Torres Chong, food photographer

Adriana Torres Chong was born in Mexico City and has worked in Mexico, France and the United States. She holds a bachelor's degree in Gastronomy from the *Universidad del Claustro de Sor Juana* in Mexico City. She has worked at highly-acclaimed restaurants, including the Au Pied de Cochon in Paris and Le Cirque in Mexico City. She also worked as the head chef of Tefal-Krups-Moulinex Gourmet

Center, a training center showcasing a variety of kitchenware. Currently, Chong lives in Honolulu where she combines her two passions—teaching Mexican cuisine at the University of Hawaii's Culinary Institute of the Pacific at Kapi'olani Community College and free-lancing as a food photographer. Her photos have been featured in the United States and abroad. Her past clients include Kāhala Mandarin Oriental Hotel and Chef Mavro Restaurant. She recently became a member of Les Dames D' Escoffier International.

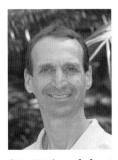

Doug Crowell, contributing author
Program Coordinator for Exercise and Sport Science
Kapi'olani Community College (KCC),
University of Hawai'i (UH).

Doug Crowell holds a master's degree in Adult Fitness and Cardiac Rehabilitation. He is a certified Personal Trainer with the National Academy of Sports Medicine (NASM) and the American Council on Exercise (ACE). He is also a certified Strength and Conditioning Specialist with the National Strength and Conditioning Association (NSCA). Crowell has done training in Mindfulness-Based Stress Reduction with the Center for Mindfulness (University of Massachusetts Memorial Health Care) and is also a certified Yoga instructor. He began his professional career as a Cardiac Rehabilitation Specialist. He has been involved in wellness education and programming for more than 20 years, in the areas of hypertension, heart disease and lifestyle management. Crowell was selected as KCC's recipient of the Board of Regents' Excellence in Teaching Award for 2004-2005.

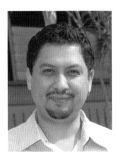

Frank M. Gonzales, editor
Non-Credit Culinary Arts Program Coordinator
Kapi'olani Community College (KCC),
University of Hawai'i (UH)

Frank Gonzales is a graduate of Stanford University with a bachelor's degree in International Relations and is a National Hispanic Merit Scholar. He also holds Associate of Science degrees in Culinary Arts and Patisserie. His responsibilities at KCC include designing and implementing public and contract culinary education and training programs. Prior to arriving in Hawai'i in 2001, he lived and worked in California's Silicon Valley as an account executive, first with

Cunningham Communications and then Blanc & Otus Public Relations. He worked with clients ranging from high tech start-up companies to Hewlett-Packard. He has also been a research analyst at the Business Intelligence Center of SRI International in Menlo Park, California, and spent several years in Washington, D.C. as a political analyst.

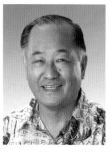

Cullen T. Hayashida, Ph.D.,
contributing author, editor
Aging and Long-term Care Training Initiative Coordinator
Kapi'olani Community College (KCC),
University of Hawai'i (UH).

Cullen Hayashida is a graduate of UH and the University of Washington (Ph.D. in Sociology). He is involved with long-term care curriculum research, and co-hosting, co-producing the Kupuna Connections TV series at KCC. He has taught at the University of Washington, Willamette University, Case Western Reserve University, and most recently at UH as a graduate affiliate faculty with Sociology, School of Nursing and the Center on Aging. His experience spans 26 years as an educator, long-term care researcher, planner, home health care director, nursing home administrator and the developer of more than 25 long-term care initiatives, in the hospital, nursing home, case management and home health care settings.

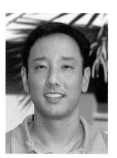

Grant Itomitsu, contributing author, editor
Registered Dietitian and instructor
Kapi'olani Community College (KCC),
University of Hawai'i (UH).

Grant Itomitsu holds a Bachelor of Science degree in the field of Food Science and Human Nutrition from UH. He has vast experience working as a clinical dietitian and educator in multiple facilities, including Kamehameha Schools, Kuakini Medical Center, St. Francis Medical Center, St. Francis Homecare, Straub Hospital, Hale Nani and Avalon Nursing facilities. Through working in multiple areas of nutrition, such as food service, clinical nutrition and education, he has gained personal insight and unique perspective in Hawai'i's diverse population. He adheres to the principle that diets are not temporary quick fixes but a perpetual investment in safeguarding a person's quality of life.

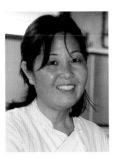

Sharon Kobayashi, contributing chef author
Chef owner
Latitude 22, LLC

Sharon Kobayashi holds a bachelor's degree in Zoology and a master's degree in Evolutionary Ecology and Conservation Biology from the University of Hawai'i. She also studied biology at the University of Washington and Cornell University, and was a biologist for the federal government. Sharon has an associate's degree in Culinary Arts from the Culinary Institute of the Pacific at Kapi'olani Community College. She has worked in restaurants in Hawai'i, Washington and California. Her professional culinary experience includes French, Pacific Rim, Japanese fusion, vegan and raw foods. She translates her eclectic experiences and interests in nutrition science and the culinary arts into product development for her business, Latitude 22. Latitude 22, dba Akamai Foods, specializes in global cuisine with a healthy flair. Their signature product, low-fat oatcakes, can be found in stores throughout Hawai'i.

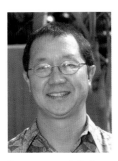

Daniel Leung, contributing author, editor
Educational Specialist
Culinary Institute of the Pacific at Kapi'olani Community College (KCC), University of Hawai'i (UH).

Daniel Leung holds a master's degree in Social Work from UH and an associate's degree in Culinary Arts from KCC. He is an alumnus of the East West Center's Institute of Culture and Communication. His responsibilities at KCC include coordinating agritourism programs, health and wellness culinary education programs and international culinary education tours. He is also an instructor for Chinese cuisine classes for the continuing education programs. Leung was a program administrator in human services for 15 years, with experience in program development and management of cross-cultural and international programs in Australia, Hong Kong and Hawai'i.

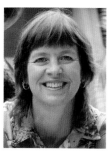

Alyssa Moreau, contributing chef author
Chef owner
Divine Creations

Alyssa Moreau has been a personal chef for private
households since 2000, focusing on healthy vegetarian
meals. Prior to that she worked with naturopathic physician Dr. Laurie Steelsmith as a dietary counselor for
patients with various health challenges such as food allergies, diabetes, heart
disease, cancer, weight loss/gain, She also worked with a computer-assisted
analysis program monitoring personal diets. Graduating from the University
of Hawaii with B.A. in Environmental Health, she worked in the local restaurant industry for over 15 years. Moreau offers private cooking lessons
and caters for small parties. She has conducted cooking demonstrations for
the Vegetarian Society as well as other private organizations. She has taught
Vegetarian/Wellness Cooking Classes for the continuing education programs
at KCC since 2002.

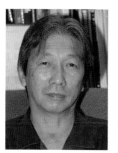

Ronald K. Takahashi M.B.A., CHE, CFBE,
principal investigator, editor
Culinary Arts Department Chairperson
Culinary Institute of the Pacific at Kapiʻolani Community
College (KCC), University of Hawaiʻi (UH).

Ronald Takahashi is a tenured associate professor and
department chair at KCC. He has a total of more than 40
years of professional and academic experience in the business aspects of both
the culinary and hospitality industries. His professional experience includes
having owned and/or operated a wide range of food and beverage opera-
tions for both hotels and independent restaurants, located in Hawaiʻi and
California. He has also been entrepreneur in the visitor industry, having initi-
ated a new concept in water sports activities on Oʻahu. Along with teaching
courses in Hospitality Purchasing & Cost Control, he has also taught classes
in Dining Room Service, Food Service Supervision, Menu Merchandising,
Equipment Layout and Design and the Hospitality Industry. 🍅

Photo Credits

Olivier Koning: KCC Culinary Arts classes 10, 11

Adriana Torres Chong: Prepared dishes and ingredients 12, 17, 23, 45, 46, 49-147, 180, front and back covers

iStockphoto: Editorial photos 14, 16, 17 (steps), 18, 20, 25, 28, 31, 32, 38, 39, 40, 42, 43, 148, 156

Daniel Leung: Island farms and farm vegetables 4, 6, 15, 17, 154, back cover; physical activities 33, 161

Kapiʻolani Community College: Culinary students in herb garden 6; physical exercises 162, 163, 164

Ed Quinto, KCC: Seniors exercising 150

Gene Phillips, KCC: Stretching and indoor bicycling 163, 164

Randall Chung, KCC: Resistance training 162

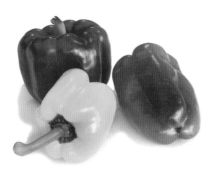